Protect Your Sight
How to Save Your Vision in the Epidemic of Macular Degeneration

by

James C. Folk, MD
Professor of Ophthalmology

and

Mark E. Wilkinson, OD
Associate Professor of Clinical
Ophthalmology

The University of Iowa
Department of Ophthalmology
& Visual Sciences

Edited by Mary Allen

Copyediting and typesetting by Patricia Duffel
Cover Design by Daniel Hunt, www.sidekick-design.com

Protect Your Sight How to Save Your Vision in the Epidemic of
Macular Degeneration

By James C. Folk, MD and Mark E. Wilkinson, OD

Published and distributed by F.E.P. International, Inc.
www.fepint.org
www.medrounds.org/protect-your-sight/

Printed in the United States of America.

For information write F.E.P. International, Inc.
941 25th Avenue, #101
Coralville, IA 52241

ISBN 0-9769689-0-8

About the Authors

Dr. James Folk is a Professor in the Department of Ophthalmology and Visual Sciences at The University of Iowa and a graduate of the Iowa Summer Writer's Workshop. He is a world renowned clinician, educator, and researcher in the field of age-related macular degeneration and has written over 125 scientific papers and books. Dr. Mark Wilkinson is an associate professor in the same department. He is secretary of the Executive Committee of the American Optometric Association's Low Vision Rehabilitation Section. He has published extensively and spoken all over the globe concerning issues related to visual rehabilitation. Together, Drs. Folk and Wilkinson provide current information about the diagnosis, treatment and management of macular degeneration.

We thank our colleagues at The University of Iowa: Michael Abramoff, H. Culver Boldt, Terry Braun, John Fingert, Michael Grassi, Thomas Casavant, Karen M. Gehrs, Greg Hageman, Robert Mullins, Stephen R. Russell, Todd Scheetz, Edwin M. Stone and Thomas A. Weingeist. Please visit us at our websites for more information:
http://www.c4md.org/or http://www.medrounds.org/amd/

We thank Patricia Duffel and Ramona Weber for their help with the manuscript. Michael L Klein MD, Professor of Ophthalmology and Director, Macular Degeneration Center, Casey Eye Institute, Oregon Health & Science University reviewed the manuscript and made many helpful suggestions.

To our families and to those who suffer
from age-related macular degeneration.

Table of Contents

Introduction –
Why You and Your Children Should Buy this Book

Let's say you've been diagnosed with age-related macular degeneration. Your eye doctor spent five minutes with you. You would like to have talked to him longer but you know how busy he is. And you were in shock when he told you your vision was probably going to get worse and that your children might get the disease too. Your mind was racing by then and you can't really remember what he said.

So what do you do next? Where do you go now for more information? To the internet? The net is jammed with advertisements for nutritional supplements and treatments that someone wants to sell you. The treatment of AMD is big business. How can you tell what claims are the truth – backed by real scientific studies – and what claims are just advertising?

How about what you read in the newspaper or hear on television? The media loves news about treatments for this blinding disease and will pretty much print anything anyone tells them about a new or miracle treatment. Journalists are not scientists and can only write what others tell them. Some experts are even paid by drug companies to promote certain treatments.

Maybe you should search the medical and scientific journals? These are better, but the articles are complicated and written for other scientists. Each paper discusses one small aspect of AMD or one new scientific finding. Even if you could understand these scientific papers, it would be hard to see the big picture.

So why is this book any different? It's different because we have written it for you, the person with age-related macular degeneration, and for people who are at risk of getting AMD. And because we're experts in this field and we're not being paid by anyone to recommend anything. We treat patients with age-related macular degeneration almost every day. We perform research that explores the causes of AMD. We attend scientific meetings. We participate in treatment trials. And we promise to tell you the straight scoop. We'll tell you what scientists and doctors all over the world know about this disease, and, just as importantly, what they don't know. The first three chapters describe AMD along with the latest science which yields clues to what causes it. You need to understand the disease in order to fight it. The last six chapters tell how you can fight back to save your vision. We will talk about changing your lifestyle, eating the right foods, and taking multivitamins with zinc along with other medications which may reduce the risk of vision loss. We will discuss the latest treatments for the wet form of AMD, including new ones that have not yet been approved but show promise. We will also talk about how to maximize your remaining vision and live as full a life as possible.

You can fight back to save your sight. We'll tell you how.

Chapter One
A Description of Age-Related Macular Degeneration (AMD)

Her name is Anna and her story is sad but familiar to those of us who work as eye doctors. She's sixty-five and has just retired. She has watched her diet, even eaten those dry, low-fat bran muffins with high fiber every morning. Her blood pressure is good, her blood lipids are way down, and she's in terrific shape. No wonder, with the yoga and step aerobic classes and all of that walking. She uses sunscreen every day. She doesn't smoke. She drinks a few glasses of wine a week but now they say that's good for you. Her PAP smears and mammograms have been A-okay. She's in the clear. Now that she's retired it's time for her to enjoy life, to do whatever she wants for the next twenty years – travel, garden, baby-sit for her grandchildren and watch them grow-up, pass her hard-earned knowledge on to them.

Then she notices that her vision is a little blurry and the straight edge of the window frame in her kitchen looks like it's bent in the middle. This is the first sign of a leak. Then the dam breaks and her vision gets worse fast. The eye doctor tells her she has the wet form of macular degeneration and that her vision is likely to get worse. She has signs of macular degeneration in the other eye too. She asks how long her vision will last, says that she loves books and needs to be able to drive to keep her independence. Her doctor shakes his head and tells her he'll do what he can.

Unfortunately, Anna's case is not unique. The western world is facing an epidemic of blindness caused by age-related macular degeneration (AMD). Unless we do something about it, this epidemic will worsen as our population lives longer. The risk of AMD skyrockets with advancing age. Seven percent of white Americans age sixty-five to seventy already have retinal changes that are known to lead to advanced AMD. Fifteen percent of white Americans have the disease by the age of seventy-five, and thirty percent have it by age eighty. There are 1.75 million people in the United States who now have advanced AMD and this number will increase to three million by the year 2020. Worse yet, the children of these people are at risk too.

So what is this disease called age-related macular degeneration, or AMD? In order to understand the disease and how it affects our vision, it's necessary to know some basic information about the structure and function of the eye. Eye doctors often compare the eye to a camera. The eye's focusing system – the cornea and lens – are like the lens in the camera. If the cornea and lens don't focus per-fectly, eyeglasses or contact lenses are used to focus the images on the eye's retina. The retina is like the film in a camera, absorbing light and converting it to chemical signals which travel to the brain. If the retina (or film) is bad, the picture you see will be too.

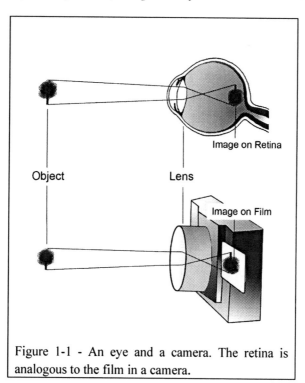

Figure 1-1 - An eye and a camera. The retina is analogous to the film in a camera.

The micro-anatomy of the eye and drusen

The eye contains two specialized receptors that absorb light and convert it to a neurochemical signal that is passed back up through the retina and onto the brain. One type of photoreceptor is called a rod. Rod photoreceptors are used for peripheral vision and for seeing at low levels of light. The other type of photoreceptor is called a cone. Cone cells work at higher levels of light and provide detailed and color vision. The macula is an area of the central retina that is loaded with cone cells. And the macula is the part of the retina we use for fine or detailed vision. The macula is the part of the retina that is most affected by age-related macular degeneration.

This process of absorbing light and converting it to a neuro-chemical signal uses up the outer part of the cone cells, called discs, and more of them have to be made every day. The cone cells rest on a layer of cells, the retinal pigment epithelium, or RPE (Figure 1-2). The RPE cells perform this yeoman's task of replenishing the discs used up by the cone cells every day. The RPE layer in turn rests on Bruch's membrane, a thin multilayered tissue which separates the RPE from the choroid, or the middle layer of the eye. The choroid is rich in blood vessels similar to a gushing river of blood. Bruch's membrane and the RPE separate this roiling river from the delicate cone cells. Necessary nutrients from the choroid cross through Bruch's membrane, are picked up by the RPE, and fed to the cones to make the outer discs that absorb light.

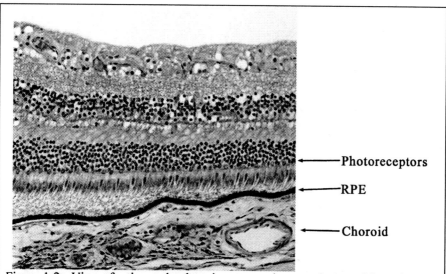

Figure 1-2 - View of retina under the microscope- the outer layers of the retina that are important in AMD are labeled

Normally the macula has a slighter darker color in the center because of more pigment in the RPE. The center may also have a yellowish color because of the luteal pigment in the inner layers of the retina. The luteal pigment protects the center from light damage and will be discussed in later chapters.

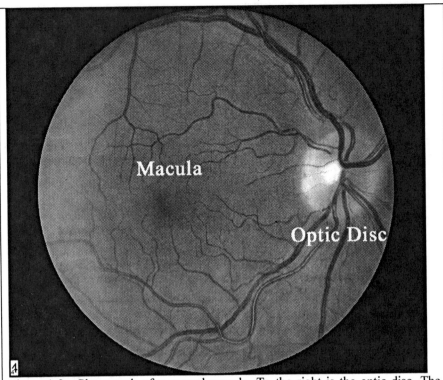

Figure 1-3 - Photograph of a normal macula. To the right is the optic disc. The center of the macula is just to the left of center and has a darker appearance.

If you have AMD, when an eye doctor looks into your eye with a special instrument, he will see round collections of yellow matter beneath the retinal pigment epithelium in your macula. These collections are called drusen (or singular, druse), a German word for stone, so named because they look like little round pebbles. The eye doctor may see only a few drusen or he may see many. In general, eyes with more drusen have a worse prognosis than eyes with fewer drusen. The eye doctor may see large drusen or tiny ones. Studies have shown that eyes with large drusen go on to develop severe AMD with vision loss much more often than eyes with small drusen. The size of the drusen is a more important prognostic sign than the number of drusen.

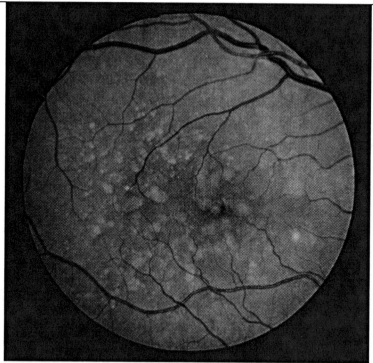

Figure 1-4 - Photograph of a macula with large, medium, and small drusen.

The eye doctor may see these drusen in your eye before you notice anything wrong with your vision. How can this be? The human body contains extra supplies of cells and sometimes even extra whole organs as backups. For instance, we have two kidneys and only really need one; there are so many cells in the lungs that smokers can kill off a lot of lung tissue before they become short of breath. Eyes with drusen have fewer cone cells or ones that are not working well, but there are enough extra cones in the macula that you don't notice anything is wrong at first.

Scientists have asked patients with AMD to donate their eyes when they pass on so more can be learned about the disease. Many generous patients have done just that. When we look at an eye with AMD under the microscope, we see lumps of material located between Bruch's membrane and the RPE. These lumps are the yellow drusen that the eye doctor sees when he looks into your eye. The abnormal material is made up of many different kinds of chemicals and

6

cellular components, so drusen have been compared to a trash heap. Scientists believe that this material probably impedes the transportation of nutrients from the blood vessels in the choroid, across Bruch's membrane, into the RPE, and then finally to the cone cells in the retina, and that it impedes the elimination of waste products from the cone cells back into the choroidal blood vessels. Perhaps drusen are the accumulated waste products that cannot get through Bruch's membrane. This blockage may cause the cone cells in the retina to get sick and die.

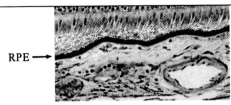 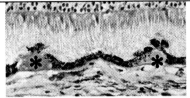

Figure 1-5A - Normal outer retina under microscope. Note RPE right on top of Bruch's membrane	Figure 1-5B - Retina with AMD under microscope. Note drusen (*) between RPE and Bruch's membrane

If you're worried that you have macular degeneration, you should ask your doctor whether he sees drusen in your eyes. Doctors don't like to give bad news so you may need to ask him or her specific questions: Does he or she see drusen in your eyes? Are they large or small drusen? How many drusen are there? The best answer your doctor can give you is that he sees no drusen. The next best answer is that he sees only a few small drusen. The presence of a few small drusen does not necessarily indicate that you have AMD. Lots of small drusen are more worrisome but even people who have these seem to stay stable for many years. If large drusen are present, though, you probably have the early stages of AMD.

Doctors divide patients into groups based on whether they have "dry" or "wet" AMD. Dry AMD basically means that there are no abnormal blood vessels beneath the retina, whereas wet, or neovascular, AMD means that these abnormal blood vessels are present.

Dry and wet AMD are not mutually exclusive. A patient can have dry AMD and then develop the new blood vessels, which means that he or she now has wet AMD.

Dry AMD

An eye with more than a few medium-size drusen or one large drusen has dry AMD. Doctors can't be sure whether patients with only small drusen or a few medium-sized drusen have the disease or not. Let's say you have some large drusen. What's going to happen to you over the next five or ten years? The appearance of your drusen may stay the same for years and your vision may remain very good. But usually your drusen will eventually change in appearance. They may enlarge or merge with other drusen. When drusen coalesce, it's usually a sign that the disease is progressing (also see Chapter Eight).

Patients who have dry AMD can lose vision by developing what is called atrophy. Atrophy means a loss of tissue. In this case, that atrophy is in the cone cells of the retina and in the retinal pigment epithelial (RPE) cells beneath them. Patients who have AMD with atrophy are more common than patients who have the wet form of the disease. With atrophy, the drusen gradually disappear, leaving behind round areas where the cone cells and RPE cells have died. The eye doctor will look into your eye and notice round areas where he can see right down to the large vessels of the choroid. Usually, the large vessels of the choroid are not usually visible because they are covered by cone cells, the RPE, and the small vessels of the choroid, but in areas of atrophy these layers are very thin or even gone. Researchers have used microscopes to examine eyes donated post-mortem by patients in various stages of atrophic AMD. In these eyes, at different stages, the RPE cells thin, become depigmented, and then disappear. The cone cells are shortened at first and then they disappear too, followed by the layer of capillaries in the choroid.

The atrophy can progress, but usually it does so very slowly. The round areas coalesce or merge, forming various shapes. Eyes with larger areas of atrophy are described as having geographic atrophy of the RPE. Luckily, the atrophy often first occurs around or away from the very center of the macula, sparing central vision. In this case, you may still be able to see 20/20 or 20/30, but you'll notice that your vision isn't as good as it used to be and that you need more light to read. There will be blank spots in your central vision which correspond to the areas of atrophy. These blank spots are called scotomata.

The doctor may see two signs in your retina which indicate that you'll probably lose more vision. The first sign is when many drusen merge into one area of yellow material. This is called a "retinal pigment epithelial detachment," because the abnormal material separates or detaches the RPE from the underlying Bruch's membrane. Retinal pigment epithelial detachments are a sign of severe disease, and when they are present, usually large areas of atrophy or new blood vessels (see below) will develop within a few years, causing vision loss. The other bad sign is when the eye doctor sees round clumps or jagged lines of dark pigmentation lying on top of the drusen in your macula. Most eyes with pigmentation develop atrophy or the wet form of the disease.

With dry AMD, it often takes years to go from 20/20 vision to, say, 20/40 vision. When your vision reaches 20/40 in your better eye, you'll be having problems seeing road signs or your golf ball or the printing in a book or newspaper. Most patients at 20/40 are able to read using magnifying glasses or hand magnifiers and can still see well enough to drive a car. But within a year or two the vision loss may accelerate and you may go from 20/40 to 20/80 or even to 20/200 vision. Even with 20/200 vision, most patients are still able to read using strong magnification, although now they sometimes need electronic magnifiers that enlarge the print and show it on a computer screen. The peripheral vision is almost never affected in patients with dry AMD.

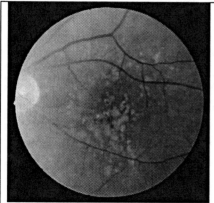 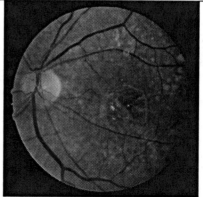

| Figure 1-6A- Eye with large drusen and pigmentation which are risk factors for progression to severe AMD | Figure 1-6B- Same eye seven years later. Now there is atrophy in center of macula making the large choroidal vessels visible |

Wet AMD

A person has wet AMD when abnormal blood vessels develop beneath the retina. Dry and wet AMD are not mutually exclusive. It is not know precisely how many people with drusen develop wet AMD but it's probably less than ten percent. The abnormal blood vessels can form in eyes with only a few drusen but in general, the more drusen you have, the greater the risk of developing new blood vessels.

The abnormal blood vessels involved in wet AMD grow from the choroid inward, through Bruch's membrane, beneath the RPE, and even through the RPE and under the fragile cone cells. These blood vessels leak fluid and bleed, which is why this type of AMD is called "wet". The blood vessels cause scarring and separate the RPE and photoreceptors from the nourishing choroid. They cause swelling in all layers of the retina, and this swelling results in distorted vision.

Distortion of Vision and the Amsler Grid

At the beginning of this chapter, Anna had developed abnormal blood vessels, and the fluid beneath her retina was causing the straight edge of the window frame to look bent and distorted. Eye doctors want people to be able to detect this distorted vision as soon as possible. The earlier it's detected, the likelier it is that the abnormal blood vessels will be small and more easily treated, with better results for the vision. That's why, if you have any signs of AMD, your eye doctor will give you an Amsler grid to take home so you can monitor your own vision. The grid looks like a miniature checkerboard and will allow you to check for any distorted vision or blind spots which may indicate abnormal blood vessels (Figure 1-7A). Most eye doctors will tell you to test your eyes with the Amsler grid every day. You should test each eye separately by covering the other eye, then focusing on the central dot of the Amsler grid. While you're looking at the central dot, you should consider whether any of the lines are missing and, more importantly, whether any of them are bent or distorted. Bent or distorted lines may mean there's fluid under your retina.

Some patients find that the Amsler grid is hard to use. They prefer picking out a calendar or a fence row or anything with straight lines to check their vision. It probably doesn't matter what you use as long as you check your vision daily and cover each eye in turn. If you don't cover each eye you may miss distorted vision, because the good eye takes over, so to speak. Researchers are developing more sensitive methods for patients to detect distorted vision earlier but these methods aren't quite ready for home use.

If you notice distorted lines, be sure to call your eye doctor within a few days rather than wait. Sometimes the technician or secretary who answers the doctor's phone won't realize the seriousness of your symptoms. She may try to put you off and give you an appointment to see the doctor in a month. It's important to be firm and demand an appointment within a few days. If the doctor is on vacation you should ask who's taking calls for him or her.

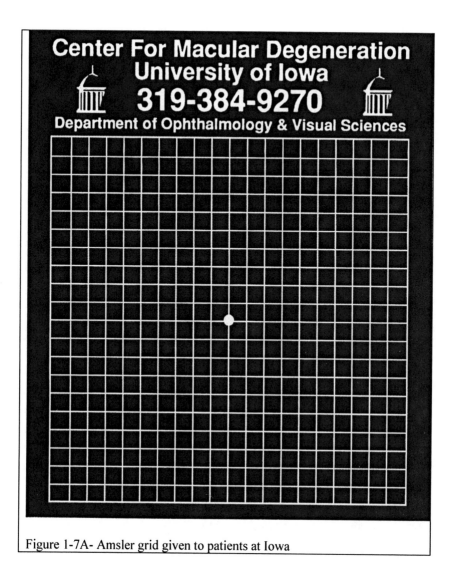

Figure 1-7A- Amsler grid given to patients at Iowa

AMSLER GRID TESTING

Purpose: To test central (reading) vision for early signs of retinal disease which may be treatable.

Directions:

1. Look through your reading glasses or bifocals.
2. Hold the grid about 12 inches from the eye.
3. Keep both eyes open and look at the dot in the center of the grid.
4. Cover the left eye. While looking at the dot, answer the following questions:

    a. Can you see all four corners of the grid?

    b. Are any of the lines: Blurry?

                                  Wavy?

                                  Distorted?

                                  Bent?

                                  Gray?

                                  Missing?

5. Repeat step 4, covering the right eye.
6. If you note any changes in how you see the grid, call your ophthalmologist.
7. We recommend you use the grid 2-3 times a week.
8. Place the grid in a convenient place which will remind you to use it regularly (for example, the refrigerator door or bathroom mirror).

The University of Iowa Hospitals & Clinics

Department of Ophthalmology may be reached by calling:

Daytime:	319/356-2215
Appointments:	319/356-2852
After 5:00 p.m., weekends and holidays:	319/356-1616

and asking for the Eye Doctor on call.

Figure 1-7B- Instructions for the use of Amsler grid

Fluorescein Angiography

At your examination, if the doctor suspects that you have abnormal vessels, he or she will ask you to have a fluorescein angiogram. A fluorescein angiogram is generally a very safe procedure, although a few patients may feel nauseated or get hives which are easily treated. Fluorescein is a molecule that fluoresces, or glows, when it's stimulated by a certain wavelength of light. During a fluorescein angiogram, fluorescein is diluted in a solution and injected into a vein in your arm or hand. From there it circulates up through the vein, into the heart, the lung, back to the heart, and then finally into the arteries all over your body. It takes about twelve seconds for the dye to make this trip before it shows up in the arteries of the eye. As the dye fills the blood vessels in your eye, a camera outfitted with special filters is used to take photographs. The images are either stored on regular film or digitally on a computer. Your doctor then studies these images. The fluorescein dye clearly shows the normal blood vessels in your eyes as well as any abnormal ones caused by AMD.

Even if you have distorted vision, you may not have abnormal blood vessels in your eyes. Sometimes patients with the dry form of AMD have distorted vision, probably because the retina has an irregular surface caused by raised areas of drusen and depressed areas of atrophy. The doctor should make absolutely sure, though, that there are no new blood vessels. If there is any doubt, he or she should see you again in a few weeks or any time your vision changes for the worse.

If you see something wrong, please don't wait. The blood vessels themselves, along with the fluid, the blood, and the secondary scarring, all cause vision loss. If the blood vessels aren't treated, they usually grow and cause a large scar in the macula, resulting in permanent vision loss. And now there are good treatments which can stop the new blood vessels.

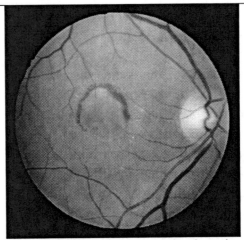

Figure 1-8A- Photograph of the macula of a patient with wet AMD showing abnormal vessels rimmed by blood.

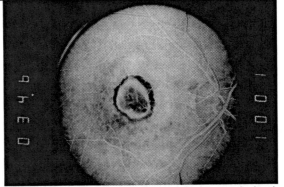

Figure 1-8B- FFA showing filling of neovascularization with fluorescein dye.

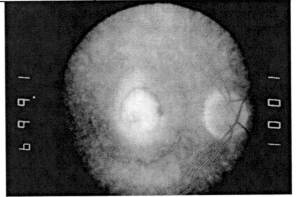

Figure 1-8C- Fluorescein dye leaks from neovascular vessels late in FFA.

Summary

Two million people in the United States now have vision loss from AMD and that number will increase as our population ages. Millions more already show signs of AMD and are at risk for vision loss in the future. AMD is a disease of the eye's outer retina and inner choroid, specifically, the layers of the cone cells, the retinal pigment epithelium, Bruch's membrane, and the inner capillaries of the choroid. There are both "dry" and "wet" forms of AMD. The first sign of AMD is drusen, which are seen by your eye doctor as yellow nodules beneath the retina. If your doctor tells you that he sees only a few small drusen, you may not even have AMD. Certainly, you have an excellent chance of seeing for many years. If he sees many medium-sized drusen or one large drusen, you probably do have early AMD. You may still see well for years, but you're at risk of developing atrophy which is slowly progressive. You're also at risk of developing new blood vessels beneath the retina, in which case you will have wet, or neovascular, AMD. A symptom of new blood vessels is blurred or distorted vision. If you notice a change in your vision, you should see your eye doctor right away. There are many new treatments for these new blood vessels, but all of them work best if they're used early when the abnormal blood vessels are small and haven't caused scarring.

A Final Word

AMD is a serious disease, but there's hope. The next two chapters will tell you more about the disease. This information is crucial, because it's important to understand AMD in order to be able to fight it. Then, in the rest of the book, we'll tell you what you can do to slow down or maybe even stop the loss of your vision, as well as how to live a full life with the vision you have.

References – Chapter One

Age-Related Eye Disease Study Research Group. AREDS Report No. 8: A randomized, placebo-controlled, clinical trial of high-dose supplementation with vitamins C and E, beta carotene, and zinc for age-related macular degeneration and vision loss. Arch Ophthalmol 2001; 119: 1417-1436.

Assink JJM, Klaver CCW, Houwing-Duistermaat JJ, et al. Heterogeneity of the genetic risk in age-related macular disease: a population-based familial risk study. Ophthalmology 2005; 112: 482-487.

Bressler NM. Age-related macular degeneration is *the* leading cause of blindness... JAMA 2004; 291: 1900-1901.

Bressler SB, Maguire MG, Bressler NM, Fine SL, the Macular Photocoagulation Study Group. Relationship of drusen and abnormalities of the retinal pigment epithelium to the prognosis of neovascular macular degeneration. Arch Ophthalmol 1990; 108: 1442-1447.

The Eye Diseases Prevalence Research Group. Prevalence of age-related macular degeneration in the United States. Arch Ophthalmol 2004; 122: 564-572.

Gass JDM. Diseases causing choroidal exudative and hemorrhagic localized (disciform) detachment of the retina and retina pigment epithelium. In Stereoscopic Atlas of Macular Diseases: Diagnosis and Treatment. 4th ed. St. Louis, MO: Mosby; 1997: 49-285.

Klein R, Peto T, Bird A, Vannewkirk MR. The epidemiology of age-related macular degeneration. Am J Ophthalmol 2004; 137: 486-495.

The Macular Photocoagulation Study Group. Risk factors for choroidal neovascularization in the second eye of patients with juxtafoveal or subfoveal choroidal neovascularization secondary to age-related macular degeneration. Arch Ophthalmol 1997; 115: 741-747.

Seddon JM, Chen CA. The epidemiology of age-related macular degeneration. Int Ophthalmol Clin 2004; 44(4): 17-39.

Wang JJ, Foran S, Smith W, Mitchell P. Risk of age-related macular degeneration in eyes with macular drusen or hyperpigmentation: The Blue Mountains Eye Study Cohort. Arch Ophthalmol 2003; 121: 658-663.

Chapter Two
What Causes AMD?

Researchers and doctors don't yet know exactly what causes AMD, but we're getting closer. AMD is most strongly associated with age and a family history of the disease. Why does age increase the risk? The answer to that may simply be that most diseases increase as we age. It takes time for genetic or environmental factors to cause damage. It takes time for the wonderful cells in our body to wear out. A person doesn't get lung cancer after smoking one cigarette or heart disease after eating one cheeseburger. A person may have some abnormal genes and then be exposed to environmental factors that increase his or her chances of developing the condition, but it may still take seventy years for the disease to show up.

Genes and Inflammation

There is good evidence that there is a large genetic component to AMD. Studies have shown that the risk of AMD is much higher for people whose family members have the disease than for people who have no family history of AMD. Identical twins, who share the same genes, often have similar features of age-related macular degeneration. Abnormalities in the fibulin 5 and 6 genes, which code for structural proteins that are found in and around the outer parts of the retina and choroid, have recently been shown to be associated with AMD in some families.

Researchers are working very hard to find more genes associated with AMD. Finding the genes is difficult, though, because macular degeneration is probably not a single disease and the changes we see in the retina, namely the drusen, atrophy, and neovascularization, can probably be caused by the interaction of a lot of different genes with many different environmental factors.

Recently, genetic studies show that variants of a protein that normally keeps inflammation in check increases the risk of AMD. This protein is called complement factor H and when modified can allow overactive inflammation. Smoking also inhibits factor H activity which may be one of the reasons that smoking increases the risk of vision loss in AMD. An additional study showed that it may be the interaction of different proteins in this complement pathway which may increase or decrease the risk of AMD.

Separate studies have shown that a mutation in the Toll-like receptor gene is associated with AMD. Toll-like receptors are involved with macrophages (a white blood cell) and the removal of foreign matter in the body. This receptor may also be involved in the removal of old outer segments in the cone cells so that they can be renewed.

Other studies also support that AMD is associated with overactive inflammation. Scientists have found cells called macrophages and giant cells, both of which are associated with inflammation, in the outer retinas of patients with AMD. The Age-Related Eye Disease Study (AREDS) found that an elevation of C-reactive protein in the blood was associated with advanced AMD. C-reactive protein is a marker of inflammation in the body, so higher levels implicate the role of inflammation in this disease.

Inflammation is a natural part of the body's immune system. It is the body's way of responding to threats such as infections or other things which it *"perceives"* as foreign invaders. Our immune system is necessary to protect us against infection. Before hygienic measures and antibiotics, most of our ancestors died from infections that were often something as simple as an infected tooth. In the old days, the humans who had the best immune systems were the ones who were "naturally selected" to survive and reproduce. But new information indicates that an overactive immune system – one which creates the most inflammation when the body *"perceives"* an enemy – causes problems later in life. Not only AMD, but also Alzheimer's disease and heart disease are now thought to involve inflammatory components. Future studies may test whether anti-inflammatory drugs should be used to treat AMD.

Later in this book, we'll recommend things you should do right now, dietary and lifestyle changes as well as which supplements to take, to curb inflammation and slow down vision loss from AMD.

Light Damage

Another theory is that chronic light damage to the retina causes AMD. When light reacts with oxygen molecules, reactive oxygen species form. These reactive oxygen species are toxic to cells, especially to the lipids in the cell walls. The outer retina and RPE have a lot of oxygen from the blood-rich choroid. These layers are also exposed to a lot of light because their job is to absorb light and start the process of vision. This combination of a lot of oxygen and a lot of light adds up to a lot of damaging reactive oxygen which may lead to AMD. Epidemiological studies, however, show variable results relating the amount of light exposure to the risk of AMD. Still, it seems wise to wear sunglasses and a hat with a brim to block excess sunlight that may damage your eyes. During cataract surgery, the intraocular lens that is placed in your eye is manufactured to block ultraviolet light, since ultraviolet light has the most energy and is potentially the most harmful.

Reduced Blood Flow

Another theory is that AMD is caused by decreased blood flow in the choroid layer. Patients with cardiovascular disease and those who have high levels of lipids in their blood, both of which are associated with reduced blood flow through the arteries, seem to have a higher risk of AMD. Smoking reduces blood flow and also increases the risk of AMD. It all seems to fit. However, the studies are not consistent. Some studies show that patients with cardiovascular disease have a greater risk of AMD, whereas other studies do not. Patients with AMD do have reduced blood flow in the choroid, but it's hard to determine which is the chicken and which the egg. Most of these studies measure the choroidal blood flow after AMD has already developed. We know that with AMD, cells are lost in the outer retina before the patient notices symptoms. The body doesn't waste its resources; if there are fewer cells to feed, the body will reduce the blood flow to that area. Therefore, the reduced blood flow in the choroid may be the result, rather than the cause, of AMD. Later in this book you'll find out that what is good for the heart (low fat diet, good blood pressure, and normal weight) is also good for the eye with AMD.

Thickening of Bruch's Membrane

There's also a theory that AMD is mainly due to changes wrought by aging in Bruch's membrane. The membrane is attacked by reactive oxygen molecules formed by the interaction of oxygen molecules with light. Lipids from the blood leach into the membrane and make it thick and impermeable to the flow of nutrients into the retina. This lack of nutrients and oxygen flowing across Bruch's membrane starves the RPE and the cone cells. They die and the end result is dry AMD with atrophy. Some researchers think this may also be a cause of neovascular AMD because the starving retinal cells may send out signals that they need more food and oxygen. The body's response to these signals may be the abnormal vessels that grow beneath the retina.

Summing Up the Possible Causes of AMD

The best guess at this time is that factors in all of the above theories play a role, but that none of them is the single cause – "the" cause with a capital "T" – of AMD. AMD probably involves many factors coming together to damage the eye over years. Genetic defects cause the first weakness in the system. Some possible genetic defects are so bad that the person who has them will get AMD no matter what. Other genes are not so bad. Maybe the people who have these genes must also have a bad diet, or smoke, or be exposed to a lot of sunlight before they get AMD. Or maybe to develop the disease they must have an overactive immune system that attacks the retina the moment it becomes a little abnormal. In most patients a combination of factors is what leads to the disease.

Although what we have written above may seem discouraging, it's actually good news that the disease is complicated and involves many factors. If many factors are involved, that means there may be many ways to treat AMD. We already know that you can slow the progression of AMD by eating healthy foods and taking antioxidants and zinc (see Chapter Four). We know you can reduce the amount of lipids in your blood by lowering the fat in your diet or taking special medicines. Lowering the level of inflammation in your body may also help. There are now drugs that can reduce inflammation although many of them have side-effects. But when we understand the exact mechanism of inflammation, patients with AMD may be able to take more specific drugs that target only the pathway involved in AMD and thus do not have side-effects. Understanding more about how inflammation affects AMD may also make it possible to decrease inflammation through lifestyle changes.

AMD is Probably Not a Single Disease:
Implications for Treatment

Right now, we lump all AMD patients together. However, since we know that AMD can be caused by a number of different things, combining all AMD patients into one group is like lumping all patients with cancer together to test a new therapy. We need more research to unlock the secrets of AMD. Once AMD is better understood, we'll be able to group together patients who have the same disease caused by the same factors. In various trials, some patients seem to respond miraculously to a given treatment whereas others don't seem to respond at all, so we already know that not all AMD patients are alike. In the future, we hope to be able to tell exactly what type of AMD you have, what it's caused by, and what specific treatment works best for your type of disease.

The dream, of course, is genetic therapy: Figure out what genes are bad and then replace them with good genes. This is rapidly becoming a reality in the case of some diseases, but with AMD it might not even be necessary to replace the abnormal gene once it's been discovered. Instead it might be a lot easier just to control the gene's bad effects. Say, for instance, that a genetic defect causes weak elastic tissue in Bruch's membrane so the membrane eventually breaks down, but if you take more vitamin C or zinc you can toughen up the membrane and make it last longer. You can also make sure that you're not overweight or have high lipids or high blood pressure so you don't stress the membrane. You may be able to delay the disease that way for years or even prevent it. Maybe if your children start taking preventive measures early in life, they'll never have a problem. And with new genetic findings, you'll eventually be able to find out through a simple blood test whether you're at risk of getting AMD or probably any other disease for that matter.

This is going to happen. Part of it is happening right now and there are things that you can do right now to reduce the risk of losing vision. That's why we hope you'll keep reading.

References – Chapter Two

Anderson DH, Mullins RF, Hageman GS, Johnson LV. A role for local inflammation in the formation of drusen in the aging eye. Am J Ophthalmol 2002; 134: 411-431.

Assink JJM, Klaver CCW, Houwing-Duistermaat JJ, et al. Heterogeneity of the genetic risk in age-related macular disease: a population-based familial risk study. Ophthalmology 2005; 112: 482-487.

Dastgheib K, Green WR. Granulomatous reaction to Bruch's membrane in age-related macular degeneration. Arch Ophthalmol. 1994; 112: 813-818.

Edwards AO, Ritter R III, Abel KJ, Manning A, Panhuysen C, Farrer LA. Complement Factor H polymorphism and age-related macular degeneration. Science 2005; 308: 421-424.

Gass JDM. Drusen and disciform macular detachment and degeneration. Arch Ophthalmol 1973; 90: 206-217.

Grizzard WS, Arnett D, Haag SL. Twin study of age-related macular degeneration. Ophthalmic Epidemiol 2003; 10: 315-322.

Grossniklaus HE. W. Richard Green Award Lecture. Presented at The Macula Society 28th Annual Meeting; February 24, 2005; Key Biscayne, Florida.

Hageman GS, Anderson DH, Johnson LV, et al. A common haplotype in the complement regulatory gene factor H (*HF1/CFH*) predisposes individuals to age-related macular degeneration. Proc Natl Acad Sci U S A 2005; 102: 7227-7232.

Hageman GS, Luthert PJ, Chong NHV, Johnson LV, Anderson DH, Mullins RF. An integrated hypothesis that considers drusen as biomarkers of immune-mediated processes at the RPE-Bruch's membrane interface in aging and age-related macular degeneration. Prog Retin Eye Res 2001; 20: 705-732.

Haines JL, Hauser MA, Schmidt S, et al. Complement Factor H variant increases the risk of age-related macular degeneration. Science 2005; 308: 419-421.

Jakobsdottir J, Conley YP, Weeks DE, Mah TS, Ferrell RE, Gorin MB. Susceptibility genes for age-related maculopathy on chromosome 10q26. Am J Hum Genet 2005; 77: 389-407.

Klaver CCW, Wolfs RCW, Assink JJM, van Duijn CM, Hofman A, de Jong PTVM. Genetic risk of age-related maculopathy: population-based familial aggregation study. Arch Ophthalmol 1998; 116: 1646-1651.

Klein ML, Mauldin WM, Stoumbos VD. Hereditary and age-related macular degeneration: observations in monozygotic twins. Arch Ophthalmol 1994; 112: 932-937.

Klein RJ, Zeiss C, Chew EY, et al. Complement Factor H polymorphism in age-related macular degeneration. Science 2005; 308: 385-389.

Lotery AJ, Goverdhan SV, Howell WM, Mullins RF, Hodgkins PR, Mwanza K. Association of HLA class I and class II polymorphisms with age-related macular degeneration. Presented at The Macula Society 28th Annual Meeting; February 26, 2005; Key Biscayne, Florida.

Rivera A, Fisher SA, Fritsche LG, et al. Hypothetical LOC387715 is a second major susceptibility gene for age-related macular degeneration contributing independently from complement factor H to disease risk. Hum Mol Genet. 2005; 14: 3227-3236.

Schultz DW, Klein ML, Humpert AJ, et al. Analysis of the *ARMD1* locus: evidence that a mutation in *HEMICENTIN-1* is associated with age-related macular degeneration in a large family. Hum Mol Genet 2003; 12: 3315-3323.

Seddon JM, Ajani UA, Mitchell BD. Familial aggregation of age-related maculopathy. Am J. Ophthalmol 1997; 123: 199-206.

Seddon JM, Cote J, Page WF, Aggen SH, Neale MC. The US twin study of age-related macular degeneration: relative roles of genetic and environmental influences. Arch Ophthalmol 2005; 123: 321-327.

Seddon JM, Gensler G, Milton RC, Klein ML, Rifai N. Association between C-reactive protein and age-related macular degeneration. JAMA 2004; 291: 704-710.

Stone EM, Braun TA, Russell SR, et al. Missense variations in the fibulin 5 gene and age-related macular degeneration. N. Engl J Med 2004; 351: 346-353.

Zareparsi S, Buraczynska M, Branham KEH, et al. Toll-like receptor 4 variant D299G is associated with susceptibility to age-related macular degeneration. Human Mol Genet 2005; 14: 1449-1455.

Chapter Three
Important Risk Factors in AMD

Epidemiological Studies

Two main types of studies have been used to try to determine which factors increase or decrease the risk of AMD. One type is the population-based study, in which the scientist questions and examines everyone in a given population; such a study was performed, for example, in the town of Beaver Dam, Wisconsin. The other type of study is called a case-control study, in which a group of patients with AMD is compared to a closely matched group of people who do not have AMD.

In each type of study, researchers ask each patient a number of questions about their health and habits. They then examine the patient to see if they have the disease in question – in this case AMD – or any other diseases associated with it. The researchers compare those who have AMD to those who do not. They search for differences between the two groups. For instance, if most of the patients with AMD smoke whereas most of the patients without AMD don't smoke, this is a difference or imbalance that suggests that smoking may be related to AMD. The researchers may then say that there is an association between smoking and AMD.

Even if an association is found, it does not mean this is a cause of the AMD. For instance, those who have atherosclerotic plaques on their carotid arteries seem to have an increased risk of AMD, but this does not necessarily mean that the plaques are causing the eye disease. There is more evidence that high cholesterol or systemic inflammation may be the cause of both the plaques and the AMD. Therefore, the plaques on the arteries and the eye disease are associated, but one isn't causing the other.

The study of which factors affect the presence or absence of a disease is called epidemiology. Epidemiologic studies have found that the two main risk factors for AMD are age and family history.

As we discussed in Chapter Two, AMD has a strong genetic component, but it takes a long time for these abnormal genes to cause changes in the retina and vision loss. The other genes in a person may influence the development of the disease. Some of these genes may hasten the onset of the disease, whereas others may be protective. For instance, small drusen are common in all ethnic groups, yet severe AMD with vision loss is much more common among Caucasians than African-Americans, and Hispanics have a risk somewhere between these two groups. Probably African-Americans and Hispanics have different genes than Caucasians which protect them against severe AMD, or alternatively, Caucasians have additional genes that make the disease worse.

Smoking

After genetic factors, the next most important risk factor for AMD is smoking. Most studies have shown that smokers have a two to four times greater risk of developing AMD than nonsmokers. This means a 200 to 400 percent increased chance of getting AMD among smokers. Some studies found the risk was even six or seven times higher in smokers. Smokers who have stopped have a risk somewhere between current smokers and those who never smoked. Smoking is by far the most important risk factor in AMD that can be controlled by the patient. In particular, smoking seems to increase the risk of severe forms of dry and wet AMD resulting in profound vision loss.

High Blood Pressure and Cardiovascular Disease

Hypertension (high blood pressure) is the next most significant risk factor. People with high blood pressure have a one-and-a-half to two times increased risk of AMD compared to those who don't have high blood pressure, according to most epidemiological studies.

A number of studies have looked at cardiovascular disease versus AMD, and the results of these studies have been variable. A few studies have shown that patients who have atherosclerotic plaques on the internal carotid artery or who have abdominal aortic aneurysms are at higher risk for AMD. It also seems that patients who have a high systolic blood pressure (the top number) or a high pulse pressure (the difference between the top and the bottom, or the diastolic number) have a higher risk. People with a high pulse pressure may have stiffer or harder arteries. Researchers don't believe that cardiovascular disease necessarily causes AMD. Instead, they believe that something else which is a common risk factor for both diseases, perhaps high lipid levels or inflammation, causes both the cardiovascular and eye disease.

Obesity and Inflammation

An increased body mass index (your weight compared to your height) is also associated with an increased risk of AMD. Central or truncal obesity (around your belly) may be associated with AMD at a higher rate than generalized obesity. Recent results from the Age-Related Eye Disease Study Group (AREDS) found that people who took antacids had a reduced risk of AMD, whereas people who took nonsteroidal anti-inflammatory medications such as ibuprofren had an increased risk of the atrophic form of the disease. These results need to be confirmed. And again, even if they are confirmed, we don't know which came first in the case of the anti-inflammatory medicines. Perhaps the patients who took them needed to take them because they had more inflammation in their bodies and it was the inflammation, not the medication, which increased the risk of atrophic AMD.

Sunlight

Studies on the effect of sunlight have had variable results, but most experts feel that excess exposure to sun, including lifetime exposure, may play a minor role in the development of AMD. Heavy sunlight exposure when you were young may be just as or more important than exposure that took place later in life. We recommend that not only patients with AMD but also their family members protect their eyes from sunlight with brimmed hats and sunglasses from an early age on.

Alcohol

The use of alcohol doesn't appear to increase the risk of AMD except in the case of smokers who drink a lot of alcohol. Here, there appears to be an increased risk of the severe wet form of the disease, but it's unknown whether this is due to the alcohol or the smoking or both.

AMD and Early Death

The Copenhagen City Eye Study recently found a 60 percent increased risk of death among women (but not men) with AMD compared to those who didn't have the disease. Was this due to an underlying genetic defect that perhaps affected not only the eye but also the rest of the body? Could patients with AMD have more systemic inflammation, as described in Chapter Two, and this resulted in a higher death rate? Or was it that these women, who had suffered vision loss, were depressed or prone to falls which led to their deaths? No one knows, but this finding may mean that the genetic and environmental factors that cause AMD can also cause an earlier death.

The Rotterdam Study however, found no increased risk of mortality in patients with AMD after adjusting for other risk factors such as smoking, body mass index, cholesterol level, atherosclerosis, hypertension, history of cardiovascular disease, and diabetes. These findings seem to indicate that these other risk factors increased both the mortality and AMD, and that it wasn't just the AMD alone that caused a higher risk of death.

Eye Color and Cataract Surgery

Some studies have found that AMD is more common in people who have blue eyes compared to people with brown or darker eyes. A few studies have found an increased risk of AMD in people with farsightedness (hyperopia) compared to those who are nearsighted (myopia), which could either mean that myopia protects against AMD or that farsighted people live longer than nearsighted ones.

In the past, large studies found that patients whose cataracts had been removed had a higher risk of AMD. The problem with these studies however, is that the maculas were not examined before the cataract surgery. So it was hard to tell whether the cataract surgery caused the AMD to progress or if the AMD was already there and that is why the patient went to the doctor in the first place. The doctor may have then removed the cataract in an attempt to improve the vision. A number of patients in the Age-Related Eye Disease Study (AREDS) had examinations and photographs of the maculas before cataract surgery. This study showed no association between cataract surgery and the progression of AMD. Now the best advice for an AMD patient is to have cataract surgery if it's necessary.

Summary

Aging and a person's genetic make-up appear to be the most important factors associated with AMD. Smoking increases the risk of AMD by a whopping three to four hundred percent. White people are most prone to severe AMD; Hispanics have a lower risk; and African-Americans have a very low risk of developing severe vision loss due to AMD. Hypertension increases the risk of AMD. Specific types of cardiovascular disease, including plaques on the inside of the carotid artery, abdominal aortic aneurysms, and high systolic blood pressure, appear to be associated with an increased risk of AMD. Other cardiovascular disease like strokes and heart attacks are also associated with AMD, but most experts now believe that cardiovascular disease and AMD may have a common cause but do not cause each other. Excessive exposure to sunlight may also play a role. Cataract surgery appears to be safe in eyes with AMD.

So what can we learn from all of these studies? We have learned that quitting smoking and getting your blood pressure under control are urgently important, especially if you're at risk of getting AMD. We have learned that someone at risk of AMD should also lose weight and keep their cholesterol in good control. We have learned that inflammation and hardening of the arteries probably increase the risk of both heart disease and AMD. This information provides clues about where to look for the exact causes of AMD.

In the next chapter we'll tell you how to use this information as well as the results of a large controlled trial to reduce your risk of severe AMD.

Table – Risk Factors for AMD Listed in Order of Importance

1. Age
2. Family history (genes)
3. Smoking
4. Hypertension
5. Cardiovascular disease, particularly atherosclerotic plaques on the carotid arteries, abdominal aortic aneurysms, and high pulse pressures (the difference between systolic and diastolic readings)
6. Diet and micronutrients (see next chapter)
7. Obesity
8. Sunlight

References – Chapter Three

Age-Related Eye Disease Study Research Group. Risk factors associated with age-related macular degeneration: a case-control study in the Age-Related Eye Disease Study: Age-Related Eye Disease Study Report Number 3. Ophthalmology 2000; 107: 2224-2232.

Age-Related Eye Disease Study Research Group. Risk factors for the incidence of advanced age-related macular degeneration in the Age-Related Eye Disease Study (AREDS): AREDS Report No. 19. Ophthalmology 2005; 112: 533-539.

Borger PH, van Leeuwen R, Hulsman CAA, et al. Is there a direct association between age-related eye diseases and mortality? The Rotterdam Study. Ophthalmology 2003; 110: 1292-1296.

Buch H, Vinding T, la Cour M, Jensen GB, Prause JU, Nielsen NV. Age-related maculopathy: a risk indicator for poorer survival in women. Ophthalmology 2005; 112: 305-312.

Christen WG, Glynn RJ, Manson JE, Ajani UA, Buring JE. A prospective study of cigarette smoking and risk of age-related macular degeneration in men. JAMA 1996; 276: 1147-1151.

Delcourt C, Diaz JL, Ponton-Sanchez A, Papoz L, for the POLA Study Group. Smoking and age-related macular degeneration: The POLA Study. Arch Ophthalmol 1998; 116: 1031-1035.

Hyman L, Schachat AP, He Q, Leske C, for the Age-Related Macular Degeneration Risk Factors Study Group. Hypertension, cardiovascular disease, and age-related macular degeneration. Arch Ophthalmol 2000; 117: 351-358.

Klein, R, Peto T, Bird A, Vannewkirk MR. The epidemiology of age-related macular degeneration. Am J Ophthalmol 2004; 137: 486-495.

McCarty CA, Mukesh BN, Fu CL, Mitchell P, Wang JJ, Taylor HR. Risk factors for age-related maculopathy: The Visual Impairment Project. Arch Ophthalmol 2001; 119: 1455-1462.

Seddon JM, Cote J, Davis N, Rosner B. Progression of age-related macular degeneration: association with body mass index, waist circumference, and waist-hip ratio. Arch Ophthalmol 2003; 121: 785-792.

Seddon JM, George S, Rosner B, Rifai N. Progression of age-related macular degeneration: prospective assessment of C-reactive protein, interleukin 6, and other cardiovascular biomarkers. Arch Ophthalmol 2005; 123: 774-782.

Seddon JM, Willett WC, Speizer FE, Hankinson SE. A prospective study of cigarette smoking and age-related macular degeneration in women. JAMA 1996; 276: 1141-1146.

Smith W, Mitchell P, Leeder SR. Smoking and age-related maculopathy: The Blue Mountains Eye Study. Arch Ophthalmol 1996; 114: 1518-1523.

Snow KK, Seddon JM. Do age-related macular degeneration and cardiovascular disease share common antecedents? Ophthalmic Epidemiol 1999; 6: 125-143.

Tamakoshi A, Yuzawa M, Matsui M, Uyama M, Fujiwara NK, Ohno Y, for the Research Committee on Chorioretinal Degenerations. Smoking and neovascular form of age-related macular degeneration in late middle aged males: findings from a case-control study in Japan. Br J Ophthalmol 1997; 81: 901-904.

Tomany SC, Cruickshanks KJ, Klein R, Klein BEK, Knudtson MD. Sunlight and the 10-year incidence of age-related maculopathy: The Beaver Dam Eye Study. Arch Ophthalmol 2004; 122: 750-757.

van Leeuwen R, Klaver CCW, Vingerling JR, Hofman A, de Jong PTVM. Epidemiology of age-related maculopathy: a review. Eur J Epidemiol 2003; 18: 845-854.

Vingerling JR, Hofman A, Grobbee DE, de Jong PTVM. Age-related macular degeneration and smoking: The Rotterdam Study. Arch Ophthalmol 1996; 114: 1193-1196.

Chapter Four
Lifestyle, Diet, and Micronutrients to Reduce Your Risk of Severe AMD

Smoking

You can't do much about the two main risk factors for AMD, which are your genes and your age. But you can reduce your risk of vision loss through lifestyle changes and diet. The third most important risk factor by far is smoking, and there is something you can do about that. If you smoke, you have to stop. If you don't give up smoking, it probably won't matter much if you do anything else suggested in this chapter. There are many new medications and patches which can help you stop smoking. Try using nicotine patches or gum for as short a time as possible though, since nicotine alone can cause worsening of AMD. Ask your doctor what you can do to quit smoking today.

Hypertension

Hypertension is associated with AMD so if you have high blood pressure, make sure it is very well treated. In the past, most doctors felt that high blood pressure was controlled if the systolic reading (the higher one) was less than 150 and the diastolic one (the lower one) was less than 90. The latest evidence supports even stricter guidelines for blood pressure control. We would recommend that you shoot for a systolic reading closer to 140 and a diastolic reading around 80. Blood pressure readings should be taken when you're relaxed and in a seated position. Generally, it's best to take two readings at least a few minutes apart, unless the first reading clearly shows that your blood pressure is in good control (140/80 or less).

Patients and doctors often explain elevated readings by ascribing them to "white coat hypertension," meaning that the anxiety about being in the doctor's office is causing the patient's blood pressure to go up. That's true, but only to an extent. If the doctor takes three or four readings and then assumes the lowest one is the correct reading, he or she may be under-treating your hypertension. Remember that there are many stresses during the day besides going to the doctor's office, all of which can elevate our blood pressure. Therefore, your doctor should not automatically assume that the lowest reading is the one that most accurately represents your blood pressure.

Some doctors don't treat elevated systolic blood pressure as long as the diastolic, or lower of the two readings, is within normal limits. There is more and more evidence, however, that systolic hypertension alone (without a corresponding increase in the diastolic reading) should also be treated and is associated with the progression of AMD. There is also a tendency for doctors to under-treat hypertension because the medications for it are costly and have side-effects. Your doctor may be satisfied if your readings are "pretty good" most of the time. Nevertheless, hypertension should be taken seriously and effectively treated, since it has been found to be associated with the occurrence of AMD and other health risks. You should tell your doctor that you're concerned about AMD and want to strive for strict control of your blood pressure.

Weight Loss

AMD is also associated with obesity even if one's blood pressure is normal. The latest theories implicate obesity, especially fat around the middle, with increased inflammation in the body. If possible, you should strive to reach the normal weight and fat percentage for your gender and age.

Anti-oxidant Vitamins

Now it's time to tackle the complicated subject of diet and micronutrients. Earlier we explained how oxygen molecules are stimulated by light to form toxic molecules called reactive oxygen species. These bad molecules damage all kinds of cellular structures, but they especially react with lipids in cellular membranes to the point where they can kill the cell. The macrophages in our body, which are part of our immune system, actually use reactive oxygen species to kill invading bacterial cells.

Hydrogen peroxide is one of these reactive oxygen species. If you remember how hydrogen peroxide bubbles and stings when you put it on cuts, you'll get a sense of what these molecules can do to your delicate retina. Research tells us that the outer retina is a kind of miniature battleground. The body has its own troops called antioxidants to destroy (scientists call it scavenge) the invading reactive oxygen species before they can do harm. The cells of the retina can be damaged permanently however if there are not enough antioxidants or if some genetic or environmental change causes an overwhelming number of reactive oxygen species.

Vitamins A, C, and E are considered the main antioxidants that protect the body against reactive oxygen species. Vitamin A is metabolized in the body from beta-carotene, one of the carotenoids (see Table 1). Carotenoids are a large family of pigments synthesized by plants. These pigments give the red and yellow colors to fruits and vegetables. The abundant green chlorophyll in leaves masks the bright colors of carotenoids except in autumn, when the chlorophyll disappears and the carotenoids shine through as the brilliant red and yellow colors of fall. The recommended dietary allowance of beta-carotene for the human body is about three milligrams per day. You can also get vitamin A itself from meat sources, particularly liver, where it is stored.

Vitamin C cannot be created from scratch in the body so it must be ingested in the diet. The dietary allowance recommended by the United States Department of Agriculture (USDA) is about 80 milligrams per day. Many people take more than this in supplement form, even as much as 500 milligrams a day. Vitamin C is water-soluble and isn't stored in the body to any great extent, so taking a higher dose is probably not harmful. A deficiency of this vitamin caused scurvy in sailors because they didn't have access to fresh fruit or vegetables.

Vitamin E is a fat-soluble vitamin that is available in nuts and oils. The recommended daily allowance is about 15 milligrams per day.

Metals such as zinc are used in enzymes, which help the body perform a variety of functions. If there is a deficiency of the metal, the enzymes can't work. Zinc is especially important in wound healing, and the recommended dietary allowance is 10 milligrams per day. Selenium is another metal used in the antioxidant enzyme glutathione-peroxidase. Fifty-five micrograms per day is the recommended dietary allowance.

So there is a good theoretical basis for the idea that vitamins and metals involved in anti-oxidation and wound-healing may be important in reducing the risk of damage in AMD. Early studies involving large groups of people found that those who had a diet rich in antioxidants had a lower risk of AMD compared to those who didn't. In a small study, patients with AMD who were given high doses of zinc had less vision loss on follow-up than patients who were given a placebo.

The Age-Related Eye Disease Study (AREDS)

Based on the evidence from these early studies, the National Eye Institute decided to perform a randomized, placebo-controlled trial to determine whether supplementation with vitamins or zinc reduced the progression of AMD. A randomized placebo-controlled trial is the best way to determine whether a given treatment works. Because this type of trial is so important, we will digress and tell you how it works.

In randomized, placebo-controlled studies, patients with a certain disease, in this case AMD, are first asked to join the trial. Only after a person joins the study is he or she assigned randomly to either the group being given the treatment or the group receiving a placebo. In the Age-Related Eye Disease Study, or AREDS, the patients were given pills to take. Neither the patients nor the doctor knew which pills, the vitamins or the placebo, they were taking. The patients were followed carefully to see which group did better – i.e., to see which patients had a lower risk of progressing to severe AMD with accompanying vision loss. The patients' vision was tested carefully in the same way every time and their retinas were examined and photographed. It is this careful follow-up and "masking" of both patient and doctor which makes the evidence from the Age-Related Eye Disease Study (AREDS) so powerful.

A total of 3,640 patients with various stages of AMD were randomized in the Age-Related Eye Disease Study into one of four groups: Patients in Group 1 were given antioxidants only (vitamin C, 500 mg; vitamin E, 400 IU; and beta-carotene, 15 mg); patients in Group 2 were given zinc only (80 mg) with a small amount of copper (2 mg as cupric oxide) to prevent potential anemia from copper deficiency caused by high zinc levels; patients in Group 3 were given antioxidants plus zinc and copper; and patients in Group 4 were given a placebo, which means that the tablets they took contained none of the above ingredients. Each patient took two tablets in the morning and two in the evening with food, to minimize stomach upset from the zinc. The pills were identical so there was no way for either the doctor or the patient to tell which pill the patient was taking.

The patients were examined at least once a year for an average follow-up time of just over six years, to determine which of them developed "advanced AMD" or lost vision. Advanced AMD meant that the eye had developed atrophy in the center of the macula (dry AMD) or had developed choroidal neovascularization (CNV).

The results of this large study showed that the risk of developing advanced AMD over five years was very low in patients who had small drusen or only one medium-sized drusen at the beginning of the trial. The risk of developing severe AMD over five years was much higher in the patients who, at the beginning of the study, had many medium- sized drusen, one or more large drusen, or advanced AMD in the other eye. In these more severely involved patients, the risk of developing advanced AMD was 28 percent in the placebo group, 23 percent in the antioxidant-alone group, 22 percent in the zinc-only group, and 20 percent in the antioxidant-plus-zinc group. Therefore, the patients who took both the antioxidants and zinc had the lowest risk of developing advanced AMD. Overall, the antioxidant-with-zinc group had a 25 percent reduction in the risk of developing advanced AMD over the placebo group. The bad news is that even the patients who took the antioxidants and zinc still had a 20 percent risk of developing AMD in at least one eye over a period of about five years.

The visual acuity results were similar, in that the patients who took the antioxidants plus zinc had a 27 percent lower risk of developing a loss of fifteen letters (three lines) on the visual acuity chart than the patients who took the placebo. Antioxidants plus zinc also reduced the risk of developing even more severe loss of visual acuity (six or more lines) and reduced the risk of developing poor visual acuity (worse than 20/100). They also seemed to reduce the risk of vision loss in eyes that already had advanced AMD at the beginning of the study. This has been confirmed in a later analysis. That means that even patients who already have substantial vision loss from AMD should still take these antioxidants and zinc. It seems that any way you slice the results, the patients who took the antioxidants and zinc did better than the patients who took a placebo. Some of them still got worse but not as many as in the placebo group.

The Safety of High Dose Vitamins and Minerals

Are the high doses of vitamins and zinc used in AREDS safe? In the AREDS, the regimen of antioxidants and zinc had few side-effects and no increase in hospitalization or mortality. The only difference among the supplement and placebo groups was an increase in hospitalization for genital or urinary-related problems in the zinc group. The high doses of zinc given during the study did have a tendency to increase prostate enlargement in men, but there is no evidence that zinc increases the risk of prostate cancer. There was also an increased rate of self-reported anemia (low red blood cell count) in patients in the zinc group, but there was no difference found in the hematocrit (a measurement of the proportion of red blood cells in the blood) of the patients taking the various supplements, including zinc, compared to that of those who took the placebo. Therefore, we don't know for sure if the zinc group had a greater risk of anemia.

Patients assigned to the antioxidant groups reported an increase in yellowing of the skin, probably due to the beta-carotene supplements, but this color change is thought to be harmless. There is good evidence from large studies, however, that supplementation with beta-carotene increases the risk of lung cancer in smokers. Therefore, smokers should not take beta-carotene supplements, although, of course, they should stop smoking to reduce the risk of AMD, cancer, and cardiovascular disease. It is unknown whether it's safe for former smokers to take beta-carotene, but it probably is, provided they have quit smoking permanently.

AREDS recently performed a follow-up analysis and found that patients who had advanced AMD, vision loss, cataracts, or cataract surgery had a higher mortality than those who didn't. The increased mortality, however, was not associated with any of the supplements taken by the participants in the study. In fact, patients who took zinc appeared to have a lower mortality. The AREDS research group concluded that the patients with more advanced AMD or cataracts who died probably had an underlying systemic disease (see the discussion about genes and inflammation in Chapter 2) which was the cause of the increased risk of mortality, and that the mortality appeared to have nothing to do with the supplements.

In the fall of 2004, there was a report that vitamin E supplementation may increase the risk of death from cardiovascular disease when used at high doses. In response to this report, two researchers,

Chew and Clemons, re-analyzed the data from the AREDS study as well as from other studies involving vitamin E supplementation. They found no increased risk with vitamin E supplementation at a level of 400 IU a day. In fact, in the AREDS, those taking the anti-oxidants plus zinc had a 14 percent reduction in mortality risk after an average time of six and a half years compared to the placebo group. We recommend that you don't take more than 400 IU of vitamin E a day until more is known.

In summary, the supplements used in the AREDS appear to be safe, though smokers should not take beta-carotene. Zinc increased the risk of prostate enlargement but not prostate cancer. And, finally, you probably shouldn't take more than 400 IU of vitamin E a day.

Lutein and Zeaxanthin

One of the emerging stories is the use of lutein/zeaxanthin supplements for preventing or slowing the progress of AMD. The two carotenoid pigments in the macula are lutein and zeaxanthin. These pigments give a yellow color to the center of the macula. They're present in a much higher concentration in the macula than anywhere else in the body so they must be there for a reason. Lutein and zeaxanthin protect against light damage in two ways. First, they're very efficient absorbers of blue light; blue light has the most energy in the visible spectrum and is therefore the most damaging. You could think of lutein and zeaxanthin as sun block for the macula. Second, they're also good antioxidants that, like vitamins C, A, and E, scavenge reactive oxygen molecules.

Patients with AMD have less lutein and zeaxanthin in their macula than patients without AMD, but, is this lack of pigment a cause or a result of the disease? The Age-Related Eye Disease Study ranked their study participants in five groups according to their dietary intake of lutein and zeaxanthin. The group who had the highest intake, the top twenty percent, had a forty percent reduction in the risk of both atrophic or neovascular AMD. These patients were probably the ones who had an overall healthier diet and ate all those good things like carrots and squash and spinach, so it is unknown whether it was their overall diet or just the lutein and zeaxanthin which made the difference. Smokers have less lutein and zeaxanthin pigment in their macula and some researches believe that may be one reason why smokers have an increased risk of AMD, though it's hard to be sure of this, since smoking does so many bad things to your body.

There have also been studies in which people both with AMD and without AMD have been given extra lutein and zeaxanthin. The studies showed that supplementation increases the levels of lutein and zeaxanthin in the serum, which means that the digestive system absorbs these nutrients and passes them into the blood stream. The studies have also shown that in most but not all patients, oral supplementation also increases the amount of pigment in the macula. Lutein appeared to be more effective than zeaxanthin at increasing the pigment in the macula. Thus, more lutein in the macula may protect against light damage and help scavenge reactive oxygen species, thus slowing the progression of AMD.

All of the above results have raised the idea that taking extra lutein and zeaxanthin may help reduce the progression of AMD. The supplements are formulated from ground-up marigolds, which contain a lot of lutein and zeaxanthin in their yellow flowers. These pigments can now also be synthesized chemically.

Age-Related Eyed Disease Study II – AREDS II

The National Eye Institute is choosing centers for AREDS II which will test whether supplementation with lutein and zeaxanthin slows the progression of AMD. The planned doses have been tentatively set at ten milligrams of lutein and two milligrams of zeaxanthin daily. Patients with AMD may decide that they should go ahead and take these supplements now, thinking that at least they won't be harmful. However, we don't know for sure that supplementing with these two nutrients isn't harmful. We thought beta-carotene would be helpful in smokers and then discovered that it increased the risk of lung cancer. We thought that very high doses of vitamin E might protect against heart attacks and found that the opposite may be true. For now, we would recommend that you eat foods that are high in lutein and zeaxanthin such as spinach and kale (see table for a complete list) and participate in AREDS II if possible.

Omega-3 Fatty Acids

The other emerging story is that of omega-3 poly-unsaturated fatty acids, which are found mainly in fish and nuts. There are high levels of these fatty acids in the outer retina and capillaries of the choroid. These fatty acids have anti-inflammatory properties and may be anti-angiogenic, which may mean that they protect against the formation of the new blood vessels found in the wet form of AMD. A number of studies have found a reduced risk of AMD in patients who have diets rich in omega-3 poly-unsaturated fatty acids. For instance, in the AREDS study, the group who had the highest intakes of omega-3 had a fifty percent reduction in advanced AMD compared to the group who had the lowest. It didn't take much of the omega-3 poly-unsaturated fatty acids to be effective, because the highest intake group ate only an average of one serving of broiled or baked fish a week.

The National Eye Institute's AREDS II trial will also test whether supplementation with omega-3 poly-unsaturated fats reduces the progression of AMD. Hopefully you will have the chance to become a participant in AREDS II. If not, you should eat baked or broiled fish at least one day a week. Salmon and halibut are excellent sources of omega-3 poly-unsaturated fatty acids.

Harmful Fats

The animal fat found in beef, pork, and lamb is linoleic acid, or omega-6 fatty acid. This is the bad fat and appears to increase the risk of AMD. There are also trans fats that are made by food companies to add smoothness or moistness to their food. Food companies chemically change unsaturated vegetable oils into saturated trans fats. Trans fats are so bad for you that the government now requires manufacturers to divulge the amount of them on the labels of food products. You should limit your intake of animal fat and trans fat and try to eat skinless chicken or turkey instead of red meat.

What about Getting these Supplements from Food?

Many people believe it is better to get vitamins, minerals, and nutrients from the food we eat instead of from a pill. In the table below, we have listed foods that are particularly rich in the vitamins, minerals, and nutrients that seem to help prevent or slow the progress of AMD. You can see from the table that someone can get 500 milligrams of vitamin C a day by eating lots of fruits and vegetables. It's a lot harder to get 25,000 units of beta-carotene but it's still doable by eating the right vegetables. It is much harder to take in the AREDS' doses of vitamin E and zinc in the diet. In addition, the oils that are high in vitamin E, such as sunflower, safflower, and soybean oil, are also high in omega-6 polyunsaturated fatty acids. In AMD, we are trying to increase the ratio of omega-3 to omega-6 polyunsaturated fatty acids, so this is counterproductive.

It is probably best to go ahead and take a vitamin that contains the doses used in AREDS but then also eat lots of fruits and vegetables as well as fish at least once a week. Can you overdo it though? Vitamin C is water-soluble and any excess will just be eliminated in the urine. The excess beta-carotene probably won't be a problem unless you're eating lots of pumpkin, sweet potato, carrots, or spinach. You can also use this table to see if you're getting too much of a good thing and, if so, back off a bit on the vitamins by skipping a vitamin pill every few days. If your skin turns a bright yellow, then you're probably overdoing the beta-carotene.

The table also shows that it's possible to get enough lutein/zeaxanthin just by eating colorful, especially dark green, vegetables. So lutein/zeaxanthin supplements aren't needed if you eat the vegetables listed, and you would get other nutrients and fiber by eating these vegetables as well.

The omega-3 polyunsaturated fat contained in nuts and seeds is alpha-linolenic acid (ALA) which is converted to eicosapentanenoic acid (EPA) and docosahexaenoic acid (DHA) in the body. EPA and DHA are the active beneficial forms of the omega-3 family. It takes 10 milligrams of ALA in seeds and nuts to make one milligram of EPA or DHA. Therefore, although a cup of flaxseeds contains 56 milligrams of ALA, it will make only 5.6 milligrams of EPA or DHA in the body, and that is a lot of seeds to eat. Fish already contain the active form of EPA and DHA. That is why most experts recommend eating fish at least once or twice a week. Fish is also an excellent source of protein. Some companies will try to sell you fish oil stating that there is too much mercury in fish and that their oil is pure. Personally, we would stick with the fish.

Table of Foods Rich in Nutrients that Fight AMD

Vitamin C: Recommended daily dose 60-90 mg. AREDS dose is 500 mg per day. Foods rich in vitamin C with amount in milligrams per one cup unless otherwise noted:

Fresh orange juice - 124	Grapefruit juice - 67
Broccoli - 116	Kale - 53
Brussel sprouts - 97	Green pepper (5 rings) - 45
Strawberries - 74	Tomato juice - 44

Beta-carotene: (converted to vitamin A in the body). Recommended daily requirement is 5000 IU. AREDS dose is 15 mg or around 25,000 IU. Foods rich in beta-carotene with IU per cup:

Pumpkin - 54,000	Peppers - 8,500
Sweet potato - 32,000	Cantaloupe - 6,000
Carrots - 31,000	Apricots - 3,000
Spinach - 15,000	Romaine-lettuce - 2,700

Vitamin E: Recommended minimal required daily dose is 20 mg or 30 IU. AREDS dose is 400 IU (about 268 mg). Foods rich in vitamin E with milligrams per cup or per tablespoon for oils:

Sunflower seeds - 64	Sunflower oil - 7*
Almonds - 56	Safflower oil - 5*
Peanuts - 16	Soybean oil - 5*
Spinach - 3	Olive oil - 2*
Flaxseed oil - 2	

* Unfortunately these oils are also high in omega-6 fatty acids which may not be good for patients with AMD.

Zinc: Recommended minimal daily requirement is 15 mg/day. AREDS dose is 80 mg per day. Foods rich in zinc with milligrams per cup unless otherwise noted:

Oysters (6 medium) - 76	Yogurt - 2
Turkey (dark meat) - 10	Kidney beans - 2
Chicken - 7	Brown rice - 1.2
Crab - 5 (average but varies with type of crab)	Spaghetti (whole wheat) - 1

Copper (trace element): Recommended minimal daily requirement is 2 mg. High zinc intake can cause copper deficiency, so 2 mg given in AREDS. Found in shellfish, beans, peas, whole wheat bread, and chocolate.

Lutein and Zeaxanthin (other carotenoids like beta-carotene): Daily minimal requirement unknown. Dose to be used in AREDS II tentatively set at 10 mg lutein and 2 mg zeaxanthin daily. Foods rich in lutein and zeaxanthin with milligram per cup:

Kale - 22	Spinach (raw) - 7
Turnip greens - 18	Corn - 3.0
Spinach (cooked) - 15	Peas - 2.2
Collard greens - 15	Brussel sprouts - 1

Omega-3 poly-unsaturated fatty acids: Daily minimal requirement is 1.5 grams per day according to Canadian FDA. AREDS II dose tentatively is a gram of DHA per day. Following are foods that are rich in omega-3 poly-unsaturated fatty acids with grams per cup unless otherwise noted. Remember that the fatty acids in flaxseed, flaxseed oil, and walnuts, are converted in the body to DHA and EPA in a 10:1 ratio. Therefore a cup of flaxseeds will be converted to 5.6 grams of DHA or EPA.

Flaxseeds - 56	Sardines - 3.5
Flaxseed oil - 2 grams per tablespoon	Herring - 2
Walnuts - 9	Tuna - 2
Wild salmon - 4	Halibut - 1

Statin Drugs

Statins have been shown to lower the risk of heart attack and stroke, presumably by lowering one's levels of low-density cholesterol (the bad one). Some epidemiologic studies showed that patients with AMD were less likely to be taking a statin drug to lower their cholesterol. Other studies have found that statins don't reduce the risk of AMD. Some studies have also shown that statin drugs appear to lower the risk of Alzheimer's disease. The statins that are currently on the market include atorvastatin (Lipitor), fluvstatin (Lescol), lovastatin (Mevacor), pravastatin (Pravachol), simvastatin (Zocor), and rosuvastatin (Crestor).

Statin drugs inhibit an enzyme in the liver which produces cholesterol. They also help the liver to remove cholesterol from the blood. If statins do, in fact, retard the progression of AMD, they may do so by reducing the accumulation of cholesterol in Bruch's membrane in the outer retina. But statins also appear to have some anti-inflammatory effect since they reduce the levels of C-reactive protein in the blood. C-reactive protein is a sign of inflammation in the body.

For now, it seems reasonable to take a statin drug if you have high cholesterol and a risk of AMD. The statin drugs will lower your cholesterol and reduce your risk of cardio-vascular disease. Should you take a statin drug even if your cholesterol is normal? Probably not. We still don't know for sure whether statin drugs really reduce the risk of AMD. And statin drugs can damage your liver. They can also cause muscle damage which is a rare (1 in a 1000) but serious side effect.

Often Asked Questions:

1. The AREDS recommends a high dose of vitamins and zinc. Would taking less than these amounts work?

Answer: No one knows. The AREDS dose of zinc (80mg) increases the risk of prostate enlargement and may be a little higher than necessary to slow the progression of AMD. The National Eye Institute will test whether a lower dose of zinc works to reduce the progression of AMD in AREDS II. For now we would recommend taking the doses of zinc and the vitamins that were used in the AREDS because they were proven to reduce the progression of AMD.

2. Would taking more antioxidants and zinc than used in the AREDS work even better at reducing the risk of severe AMD?

Answer: No one knows this either, but we wouldn't recommend it. The doses used in the AREDS study are relatively high already. Vitamins are drugs too and as such should be treated with respect. Vitamin E at doses of 400 IU a day appears to be safe but there may be increased mortality with megadoses of Vitamin E. Taking more of something isn't necessarily better. Two Tylenol® will get rid of your muscle aches. Twenty Tylenol® won't work any better and will give you liver damage.

3. Should I take other vitamins along with the AREDS formulation? And is it better to get these supplements through food?

Answer: If you take a multivitamin, we suggest you try to adjust the vitamins you take for your eyes so you don't go above the doses given in the AREDS, since higher doses than those in the AREDS formula are not recommended. This is less important for vitamin C because it is water soluble and excess is removed in the urine. It is probably more important for beta-carotene, vitamin E, and zinc.

It's probably always better to get your vitamins through food, but this is often impossible. If we examine the tables we see that there's a pretty good chance you could get the AREDS dose of vitamin C and maybe beta-carotene in your diet. It would be very tough, however, to get enough vitamin E or zinc.

4. Should I take vitamins if I just have a few small drusen?

Answer: Category one patients in the AREDS had only a few tiny drusen and category two patients had either multiple small drusen or a few medium-size drusen with or without pigmentation. Both of these groups had a low risk of developing AMD over the five to seven years of the study. That could mean that these patients don't have AMD, are at low risk for vision loss, and therefore don't need to take the vitamins. Or it could mean that these patients do have AMD but it is very early in the disease and the AREDS just didn't follow them long enough to detect it. Some of the category one and two patients did eventually develop advanced AMD. We also know from the AREDS study that there is a low risk of side-effects from taking the vitamin and zinc supplements, at least for up to five years. In addition, there is a principal in medicine that any prophylactic treatment is more effective if it's started earlier rather than later. For these reasons, if you have more than just a few small drusen, we recommend that you start taking the supplements, especially if you have a family history of AMD.

5. What should I do if I have a family history of macular degeneration?

Answer: You should get your eyes examined for signs of AMD such as drusen, atrophy, or hyperpigmentation. If you have any of these signs, start taking the vitamins. Often, however, there will be no signs of AMD before the age of fifty. If you have no signs of AMD but one of your parents is affected, you might start taking at least a multivitamin which has the daily recommended doses (not the high doses from AREDS) of antioxidants and zinc. Again, no one knows the answer to this question, but it seems reasonable to compromise or "split the difference," so to speak.

6. Which supplement should I take?

Answer: Food supplements, including vitamins and minerals, are not generally monitored by the Food and Drug Administration. Therefore, you have little assurance that a given tablet actually contains the amount of vitamins or zinc that it claims. Nevertheless, you should examine the labels and make sure the pills contain what the patients in the AREDS took, namely: vitamin C, 500 milligrams; vitamin E, 400 international units; beta-carotene, 15 milligrams (about 25,000 international units); zinc, 80 milligrams; and copper, 2 milligrams every day. We know that the progression of AMD was slowed with these doses.

We checked out what was available on the internet and at our local low-cost retailers like Wal-Mart and Target. The following products (with their monthly cost in parentheses) state that they contain close to the doses used in the AREDS: Visivite® ($13.95 on the internet); Viteyes® ($26.63 on the internet); Preservision Gel Tabs® ($13.98); and ICAPS® ($14.60).

Wal-Mart also markets Equate Vision Formula® which costs only $4.97 for 120 tabs. The bottle says to take one or two pills daily. Even if you took two pills a day you would only get 2000 IU of beta-carotene, or 8 percent of the dose used in AREDS; you would also get only 30 percent of the dose of Vitamin E used in AREDS. You would have to take 25 Equate Vision Formula® pills to get the AREDS dose of beta-carotene, and this would give you high and probably toxic doses of vitamin C, zinc, and vitamin E. So we don't recommend Equate Vision Formula®. A vision formula marketed by Walgreen's called Ocutabs® has the same problem and also is not recommended.

Supplements advertised by the radio commentator Paul Harvey are called Premier Formula for Ocular Nutrition®. This line of products contains close to the AREDS doses but also contains a lot of other supplements. They cost $44.95 for a 25-day supply and there is little evidence that the bilberry, selenium, or chromium in this supplement is helpful in AMD.

We discussed lutein in this chapter and how it may be helpful in patients with AMD. Some pharmaceutical companies have added lutein to their vision formulas but have in turn reduced their beta-carotene. For instance, there is ICAPS® with lutein which contains only 6,600 IU of beta-carotene. Preservision® with lutein contains no beta-carotene at all. Apparently the chemists thought the lutein would make up for the beta-carotene, but there is no evidence that this is valid. Therefore, we recommend you take one of the supplements which contain the full AREDS dose and then add an extra 10 milligrams of lutein and two milligrams of zeaxanthin daily in separate tablets.

Please also beware of vitamins that state they contain 100 percent of the minimum daily requirements. These doses – vitamin C, 60 milligrams; beta-carotene, 5000 IU; vitamin E, 30 IU; and zinc, 15 milligrams – are far below those used in AREDS. Patients with AMD may need far more than the 100 percent daily requirements.

We are not paid by any of the following companies. We would recommend Alcon's ICAPS® (the one without lutein) or Bausch and Lomb's Preservision Gel Tabs®, also without lutein. These supplements are sold virtually everywhere. Both of these companies are reputable and their supplements' cost is equivalent to the other. You could also consider taking the extra lutein and zeaxanthin (again, 10 milligrams of lutein and two milligrams of zeaxanthin a day), or just eat a lot of highly colored fruits and vegetables.

7. **What about the testimonials I hear on the radio or TV that say one treatment or another is the best?**

Answer: There are a number of companies that use testimonials to sell multivitamins or other treatments for AMD; the testimonials are from grateful people who regained their sight after taking the vitamin or undergoing the treatment. It's easy to be swayed by these ads because normally we trust testimonials from people like ourselves. We believe that if someone else says something worked for them, then it will work for us too. In general, however, in our opinion, these testimonials aren't worth very much. There have been excellent studies which have shown certain treatments are effective with AMD. Yet even in these studies there were many people in the placebo group who did well, so just because someone thinks a certain drug or treatment worked for them, it doesn't necessarily mean it's true. AMD is a variable disease and some people will do relatively well no matter what treatment they are given. There is also a placebo effect, wherein some people who want to get better will get better even though the treatment proves to be ineffective. That is why the best studies have control groups of patients taking placebos, to eliminate the possibility that someone's response to a given treatment is a result of this placebo effect.

If a hundred thousand people take a certain supplement or try a certain treatment, some of them are going to get better even though it may have nothing to do with the treatment. But these patients may believe that it was the treatment which caused their improvement in vision. They may be extremely grateful and write letters praising the treatment. Advertisers may then use these letters to convince you to buy their product. Please remember, though, that these letters really don't tell us anything except that one patient happened to do well. There may have been hundreds of other patients who didn't improve and didn't bother to write letters, or whose critical letters the advertisers, of course, would never use in their ads. Although this may feel counterintuitive, we caution you to avoid being swayed by testimonials. In our experience, testimonials are usually used by advertisers who want to sell you something when they really have no proof that it works. Products that do work have scientific findings to back them up and don't need such letters. Let the buyer beware.

8. What about the advertisements that say selenium, bilberry, and chromium help to reduce vision loss in AMD?

Answer: Selenium is a trace mineral that is a necessary part of an important anti-oxidant enzyme called glutathione peroxidase, which is found in the eye. A few small studies have shown that lower selenium levels are associated with AMD, and selenium is a cofactor in an anti-oxidant enzyme like the vitamins used in the AREDS. There are other larger studies t showed no relationship. Almost all Americans get the 55 micrograms daily requirement of selenium from their diet. Would taking more help? No one knows. Please remember that selenium is not a natural herbal supplement. It is a heavy metal and taking more than 400 micrograms a day of selenium is not recommended.

The notion that bilberry can be used to enhance night vision arose from anecdotal reports of British Royal Air Force aviators in World War II eating bilberry jam to improve their night vision.

Canter and Ernst identified 30 clinical trials relevant to vision in reduced light. Twelve of these studies were placebo-controlled. They found that no recent studies have shown a positive effect of bilberry on night vision or night contrast sensitivity from a high dose of bilberry taken for a significant duration. They concluded that "The hypothesis that bilberry improves normal night vision is not supported by evidence from rigorous clinical studies"

The *PDR for Herbal Medicine, Facts and Comparisons, the Review of Natural Products* and the *The Complete German Commission E Monograph: Therapeutic Guide the Herbal Medicines* lists diarrhea and inflammation of the mouth and throat as indications for the use of bilberry. There is no mention in any of these publications that bilberry is of assistance for impaired night vision. There is quite simply no evidence that bilberry helps to retard vision loss in people with AMD.

We could find no evidence in the literature that chromium retards the progression of AMD either.

Summary

The following summarizes our recommendations for what should you do if you've been diagnosed with AMD or are at risk of the disease:
1. Quit smoking. No wiggle room here. It simply must be done.
2. Control your blood pressure. A blood pressure of less than 150/90 is good. A blood pressure of 140/80 or lower is even better.
3. If you're overweight, especially around the belly, try to lose it. Strive to reach a normal weight and fat content. The ranges of normal depend on your gender, height, and age and are readily available from numerous sources.

4. Eat lots and lots of colorful fruits and vegetables.
5. Eat baked or broiled fish once or preferably twice a week. Eat walnuts and perhaps a cereal that contains crushed flax seeds.
6. Limit your intake of beef, pork, or lamb. Chicken or turkey is okay but is best with the skin removed.
7. If your cholesterol is high, ask your doctor about taking a statin drug.
8. If you have only a few small drusen or one medium-sized drusen, and no pigmentation in your retina, consider taking a one-a-day multivitamin supplement.
9. If you have many intermediate-sized drusen, any large drusen, pigmentation, or any sign of atrophy or neovascularization, take the supplements at the dosage used in the AREDS. That means 500 milligrams of Vitamin C, 400 IU of Vitamin E, 15 milligrams (about 28,000 IU) of beta-carotene, 80 milligrams of zinc as zinc oxide, and 2 milligrams of copper to prevent potential anemia. You should not take beta-carotene supplements if you smoke because of the increased risk of lung cancer. Ingesting beta-carotene in the diet by eating fruits and vegetable seems to be okay in smokers.
10. Limit your supplements of vitamin E to 400 IU a day. Many nutritional supplements, even some preparations of fish oil, have added vitamin E so it is important to add up the total amount from all sources. Don't overdo beta-carotene or zinc either. The AREDS' doses are already high.
11. As a colleague of mine tells his patients with AMD, "What's good for the heart is good for the eye." Eat healthy food with lots of vegetables, and exercise regularly.

References – Chapter Four

Age-Related Eye Disease Study Research Group. AREDS Report No. 8: A randomized, placebo-controlled, clinical trial of high-dose supplementation with vitamins C and E, beta carotene, and zinc for age-related macular degeneration and vision loss. Arch Ophthalmol 2001; 119: 1417-1436.

Albanes D, Heinonen OP, Taylor PR, et al. α-tocopherol and β-carotene supplements and lung cancer incidence in the Alpha-Tocopherol, Beta-Carotene Cancer Prevention Study: effects of baseline characteristics and study compliance. J Natl Cancer Inst 1996; 88: 1560-1570.

The Alpha-Tocopherol, Beta Carotene Cancer Prevention Study Group. The effect of vitamin E and beta carotene on the incidence of lung cancer and other cancers in male smokers. N Engl J Med 1994; 330: 1029-1035.

AREDS Research Group. Associations of mortality with ocular disorders and an intervention of high-dose antioxidants and zinc in the Age-Related Eye Disease Study. AREDS Report No 13. Arch Ophthalmol 2004; 122: 716-726.

Augustin AJ, ed. Nutrition and the Eye: Basic and Clinical Research (Developments in Ophthalmology, vol 38). Karger Publications, Basel, 2005.

Axer-Siegel R, Bourla D, Ehrlich R, et al. Association of neovascular age-related macular degeneration and hyperhomocysteinemia. Am J Ophthalmol 2004; 137: 84-89.

Beatty S, Koh HH, Phil M, Henson D, Boulton M. The role of oxidative stress in the pathogenesis of age-related macular degeneration. Surv Ophthalmol 2000; 45: 115-134.

Beatty S, Murray IJ, Henson DB, Caraden D, Koh HH, Boulton ME. Macular pigment and risk for age-related macular degeneration in subjects from a northern European population. Invest Opthalmol Vis Sci 2001; 42: 439-446.

Canter, PH, Ernst, E. Anthocyanosides of *Vaccinium myrtillus* (Bilberry) for Night Vision: A Systematic Review of Placebo-Controlled Trials .Surv Ophthalmol 2004;49: 38-50.

Chew EY, Clemons T. Vitamin E and the Age-Related Eye Disease Study supplementation for age-related macular degeneration. Arch Ophthalmol 2005; 123: 395-396.

Chew EY, Friberg T, Clemons T, Bressler S, Ferris FL, and the Age-Related Eye Disease Study (AREDS) Research Group. The effect of AREDS supplementation on visual acuity loss in eyes with advanced age-related macular degeneration (AMD). Presented at The Macula Society 28th Annual Meeting; February 24, 2005; Key Biscayne, Florida.

Cho E, Hung S, Willett WC, et al. Prospective study of dietary fat and the risk of age-related macular degeneration. Am J Clin Nutr 2001; 73: 209-218.

Eye Disease Case-Control Study Group: Antioxidant status and neovascular age-related macular degeneration. Arch Ophthalmol 1993; 111: 104-109.

The Eye Disease Case-Control Study Group: Risk factors for neovascular age-related macular degeneration. Arch Ophthalmol 1992;110: 1701-1708.

Facts and Comparisons: The Review of Natural Products. St Louis, Mo.:Wolters Kluwer, 1999.

Jarrard DF. Does zinc supplementation increase the risk of prostate cancer? Arch Ophthalmol 2005; 123: 102-103.

Klein R, Klein BEK, Tomany SC, Danforth LG, Cruickshanks KJ. Relation of statin use to the 5-year incidence and progression of age-related maculopathy. Arch Ophthalmol 2003; 121: 1151-1155.

Krinsky NI, Landrum JT, Bone RA. Bioloical mechanisms of the protective role of lutein and zeaxanthin in the eye. Annu Rev Nutr 2003; 23: 171-201.

Mares-Perlman JA, Brady WE, Klein R, et al. Serum antioxidants and age-related macular degeneration in a population-based case-control study. Arch Ophthalmol 1995; 113: 1518-1523.

Mares-Perlman JA, Millen AE, Ficek TL, Hankinson SE. The body of evidence to support a protective role for lutein and zeaxanthin in delaying chronic disease: overview. J Nutr 2002; 132: 518S-524S.

McGwin G Jr, Owsley C, Curcio CA, Crain RJ. The association between statin use and age related maculopathy. Br J Ophthalmol 2003; 87: 1121-1125.

McGwin G Jr, Xie A, Owsley C. The use of cholesterol-lowering medications and age-related macular degeneration. Ophthalmology 2005; 112: 488-494.

Newsome DA, Swartz M, Leone NC, Elston RC, Miller E. Oral zinc in macular degeneration. Arch Ophthalmol 1988; 106: 192-198.

Omenn GS, Goodman GE, Thornquist MD, et al. Risk factors for lung cancer and for intervention effects in CARET, the beta-carotene and retinol efficacy trial. J Natl Cancer Inst 1996; 88: 1550-1559.

Phelps Brown NA, Bron AJ, Harding JJ, Dewar HM. Nutrition supplements and the eye. Eye 1998; 12: 127-133.

Seddon JM, Ajani UA, Sperduto RD, et al. Dietary carotenoids, vitamins A, C, and E, and advanced age-related macular degeneration. JAMA 1994; 272: 1413-1420.

Seddon JM, Cote J, Rosner B. Progression of age-related macular degeneration: association with dietary fat, transunsaturated fat, nuts, and fish intake. Arch Ophthalmol 2003; 121: 1728-1737.

Seddon JM, Rosner B, Sperduto RD, et al. Dietary fat and risk for advanced age-related macular degeneration. Arch Ophthalmol 2001; 119: 1191-1199.

Wilson HL, Schwartz DM, Bhatt HRF, McCulloch CE, Duncan JL. Statin and aspirin therapy are associated with decreased rates of choroidal neovascularization among patients with age-related macular degeneration. Am J Ophthalmol 2004; 137: 615-624.

Chapter Five
Treatments for the Neovascular or Wet Form of AMD

Introduction

As has already been mentioned, the wet form of AMD is caused by the growth of new blood vessels beneath the retina. These blood vessels are called choroidal neovascularization because they start in the choroid and grow inward toward the retina. The abnormal blood vessels leak fluid or blood beneath and into the retina. The retina normally is smooth and flat like a mirror. When fluid accumulates under it, the vision becomes distorted. Doctors call this symptom of distorted vision, metamorphopsia. Patients may notice that the lines of objects such as telephone poles or window frames, which they know to be perfectly straight, now look bent to them. The Amsler grid, with its checkerboard pattern of lines, helps patients detect distorted vision as early as possible (see Chapter One). In addition to being distorted, the vision is usually also blurred because the retina is elevated and swollen and cannot produce a good picture to send back to the brain. Finally, a patient with wet AMD may also notice blind spots in or around the center of his or her vision. These blind spots may be due to blood or scar tissue beneath the retina.

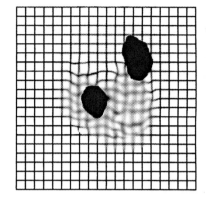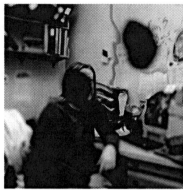

| Figure 5-1A - Amsler grid showing central distortion and scotomata (blank spots) in patient with wet AMD | Figure 5-1B - Photograph showing what patient would see. |

The body reacts to the abnormal blood vessels in AMD with inflammation. If the blood vessels are not treated, the vessels and inflammation cause a permanent scar and once the scar develops, the vision is usually damaged irrevocably. Therefore, it is urgently important to call your doctor right away if you notice any change in your vision. This is particularly true if you notice that straight lines are bent, because this may be the first sign of the abnormal blood vessels associated with wet AMD. In this chapter we'll describe treatments for these new blood vessels. All of these treatments are more effective and result in better vision if they are given early when the area of abnormal blood vessels is small and permanent scarring hasn't already taken place.

Below are descriptions of the various treatments that have been used to treat neovascular AMD. Most of them were proven to be effective through randomized controlled trials. As discussed earlier, randomized controlled trials are the best method to determine whether any given treatment is effective. In these types of trials, when patients with the disease join the trial, neither they nor their doctors know which treatment they will receive. They are then randomized by a computer to receive a given treatment. Randomization is analogous to flipping a coin.

The controlled part of the trial means that some patients will be randomized to receive no treatment. There are two potential problems that can influence the results when some patients are randomized to a treatment and others to no treatment. The first is that patients who receive a treatment may have a "placebo" effect. Patients want to get better and may think they are getting better if they're given a new treatment. The second "problem" is that some patients get better on their own whether they have treatment or not.

Both of these problems can be solved by giving the patients in the control group a placebo such as a pill or a sham treatment that should have no reason to help the condition. Now everyone in the study thinks they are getting treatment which should balance out any placebo effect. Some of these untreated patients will get better and this will give the researchers an idea how often this diseases improves without treatment. It follows then that any difference between the treatment and placebo groups should be due to the drug or the treatment.

Treatments for Neovascular AMD

Thermal Laser

Eye doctors began to understand what was happening in the wet form of AMD about thirty years ago. They followed their patients with wet AMD and saw that new blood vessels continued to grow beneath the macula until they caused a large scar. The doctors wondered if the blood vessels could be destroyed with a laser beam in order to stop their growth and spare some of the macula and central vision. Eye doctors started to perform laser treatment on the abnormal vessels in the early 1980s. They focused the laser beam carefully on the abnormal vessels. The light beam was absorbed by pigment and blood in the abnormal vessels and surrounding tissues and converted to intense heat. The heat then closed and ultimately destroyed the new blood vessels. This treatment is now called "thermal laser" because it uses an intense burn to destroy the new blood vessels (other, newer treatments using a "cold laser" are described below).

The major problem with thermal laser is that it also destroyed the normal retina in the area of the blood vessels. It is analogous to a surgeon having to destroy some of the normal surrounding tissue when removing a tumor.

Some AMD patients did well with this treatment, but it wasn't known for sure whether they were better off than if they had simply been left alone. So in the 1980s, large randomized controlled trials called the Macular Photocoagulation Studies tested whether thermal laser was better than no treatment. The studies showed that thermal laser procedures did help preserve vision. The patients who responded best to thermal laser treatments had small blood vessels that were farther away from the center of the macula. Blood vessels that were closer to the center of the macula could also be destroyed but at the cost of damaging most of the macula, which resulted in loss of vision and a blank spot in the center of the vision. The other major problem with thermal laser treatment was that the blood vessels often grew back after treatment. Perhaps this was not surprising, since nothing was really being done to treat the underlying disease. We were burning weeds, so to speak, while doing nothing to prevent them from growing right back. Another problem with thermal laser was that, since the blood vessels are not always discrete, it was tough to outline their exact extent and know where to treat and also where not to treat. The biggest problem with this treatment, though, was that it was not very effective when abnormal blood vessels were under the center of the macula. As mentioned above, these blood vessels could be destroyed with the laser, but most of the macula and central vision were lost in the process. Patients with blood vessels beneath the macula center still did slightly better in the long run after laser treatment compared to patients who were merely observed but not by much. Thermal laser is still used for small areas of blood vessels which do not extend beneath the center of the macula.

Visudyne®, or Photodynamic Treatment

A big advance in the treatment of new blood vessels in AMD occurred four years ago with the advent of Visudyne®, or photodynamic therapy (PDT). With this treatment, a special dye called verteporfin is infused into an arm vein over the course of ten minutes. The dye diffuses throughout the body and enters into the abnormal blood vessels beneath the retina. Five minutes after the last of the dye has been infused, an infrared laser set at low power is used to stimulate the dye which has accumulated in the abnormal blood vessels. The laser power is strong enough to activate the dye, which then causes damage to the abnormal blood vessels but is not strong enough to burn the overlying retina. That's why some experts call it a cold laser in distinction to thermal laser. It isn't really cold. It just doesn't heat the tissue enough to cause a burn. Visudyne® was proven to be better than no treatment in a number of large clinical trials.

Visudyne®, or PDT, treatment usually has to be repeated every three months for a total of three or four treatments until the blood vessels become "inactive." Inactive means that the blood vessels are no longer leaking, bleeding, or causing fluid beneath the retina. The treatment does not usually get rid of the blood vessels entirely. Most patients are left with scars beneath the retina which are comprised of inactive blood vessels and scar tissue.

Large randomized controlled studies have shown that, on average, patients who've had Visudyne® lose a little vision but significantly less vision than is lost by patients who have not had any treatment. On average, patients with classic choroidal neovascularization (new blood vessels that fill quickly and leak a lot on the fluorescein angiogram) lost about two lines of vision after two years of follow-up if they were treated with Visudyne®, compared to a loss of four and a half lines if they were not. Patients with occult neovascularization (new blood vessels that filled slowly on the fluorescein angiogram and leaked less) lost about three lines after two years compared to three and a half lines of loss in the group that received no treatment.

Visudyne® didn't cause the severe damage to the macula which thermal laser does. Patients who had small neovascular membranes at the beginning of the Visudyne® studies ended up with smaller scars and better vision after Visudyne® than patients who had larger neovascular membranes. Once again, this shows why it is so important for you to go to the eye doctor as soon as you notice something is wrong.

The risk of Visudyne® treatment in the studies was low. During the infusion of the drug, about two percent of patients experienced back pain which could be severe but was transient. About three percent of patients had rapid vision loss within a week after treatment; the vision loss was usually caused by bleeding or increased leakage of fluid under the retina from the abnormal blood vessels and was presumably due to the treatment. Another risk is that verteporfin sensitizes the skin to sunlight. Patients who have Visudyne® should not expose any part of their skin to direct sunlight for three days after the treatment in order to prevent severe sunburn. Sun blocks are not sufficient to protect against this, so generally the patient needs to stay in the house during the day and away from any direct sunlight even if it's coming through a window.

Otherwise the treatment is easy for patients and appears to be safe. In most patients, the treatment has to be repeated every three months for about a year so, on average, about four treatments are needed to control the blood vessels. After that series of treatments, the neovascular membrane usually, but not always, becomes inactive and stable. Visudyne® was the first good treatment for neovascular membranes in AMD that extended beneath the center of the macula. The total cost of each treatment, including the doctor's visit, is about $2500, but Medicare and most insurance carriers pay for it because it reduces vision loss in AMD.

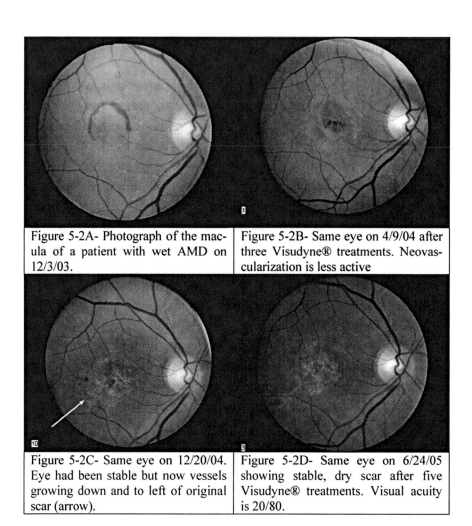

| Figure 5-2A- Photograph of the macula of a patient with wet AMD on 12/3/03. | Figure 5-2B- Same eye on 4/9/04 after three Visudyne® treatments. Neovascularization is less active |
| Figure 5-2C- Same eye on 12/20/04. Eye had been stable but now vessels growing down and to left of original scar (arrow). | Figure 5-2D- Same eye on 6/24/05 showing stable, dry scar after five Visudyne® treatments. Visual acuity is 20/80. |

Visudyne® with Intraocular Kenalog®

Visudyne® causes an inflammatory response that results in more fluid leaking under the retina for the first week after treatment. Eye doctors started to inject a corticosteroid drug into the eye after Visudyne® to blunt this inflammatory response and to try to decrease the risk of recurrent growth or leakage from the neovascular vessels. Corticosteroids are anti-inflammatory drugs like cortisone or prednisone, and do not build muscle like anabolic steroids used illegally by some athletes. The corticosteroid that is used is called Kenalog®; its generic name is triamcinolone acetonide. The drug is a white liquid designed to release slowly so that it lasts about three months after injection in the average eye and is generally very well tolerated. Multiple nonrandomized and uncontrolled studies have shown that Visudyne® with an injection of Kenalog seems to work better than Visudyne® during the first year of followup. Some studies, that have been reported but not yet published, found that after one year, patients who received both Visudyne® and Kenalog® had actually gained a line or two of vision on average, whereas patients who had Visudyne® alone had lost one or two lines of vision. Other studies have shown that after one year, patients who received both treatments did no better than patients who were treated with Visudyne® alone. The patients who received both Visudyne® and Kenalog® needed fewer treatments to control the neovascularization than patients who received Visudyne® alone.

The Kenalog® injection works best if it is given either before or immediately after the PDT treatment. The outside of the eye is numbed with an anesthetic but sometimes the patient still feels a little pain as the needle perforates the outer wall of the eye. The patient also immediately see floaters; these floaters are the white medicine floating in the vitreous inside the eye. There is a small, perhaps one in two hundred, risk of an infection in the eye after the injection. For reasons that are not well understood but probably involve changes in the drainage channels of the eye, corticosteroids can cause increased intraocular pressure, or glaucoma. The increased pressure develops in thirty percent of patients and is called a steroid response. Eye drops that are used to control glaucoma will bring the pressure down to normal levels in most patients but a few patients have needed glaucoma surgery to lower the pressure and avoid vision loss. Therefore, Kenalog® should not be used in patients who already have significant glaucoma. The exception would be if the glaucoma patient has already had an operation that controls their intraocular pressure without eye drops.

None of the studies using Kenalog® with Visudyne® were controlled or randomized, which means that none of them compared patients who received Visudyne® alone, head to head, to people who received Visudyne® plus the injection of Kenalog®. However, most eye doctors believe that, at least in the short run, the results of Visudyne® with Kenalog® are better than those of Visudyne®

alone. The positive results are probably due to the fact that the Kenalog® reduces the amount of fluid within and under the retina. In the long run, however – after two years – the final vision may be the same whether or not Kenalog® was used with Visudyne®. We should know whether Visudyne® with Kenalog® is more effective than Visudyne® alone in a year or so when large numbers of patients have been followed for a full two years. A pharmaceutical company called Novartis is also sponsoring a new randomized study that will compare Visudyne® with Kenalog® to Visudyne® with Macugen®.

Pegaptanib – Macugen®

Macugen® is a small molecule that binds to one form of vascular endothelial growth factor, or VEGF, and inactivates it. VEGF is a small protein produced by cells that are not getting enough oxygen or nutrients. VEGF is secreted by the cell, moves through the tissue, and attaches to a receptor on the outside of the endothelial cells which line the walls of blood vessels. VEGF causes the blood vessels to leak and also causes new blood vessels to grow. A lot is known about VEGF because of cancer research. Cancer cells produce VEGF in order to stimulate the formation of new blood vessels to feed the growing tumor. Scientists have long believed that if there were some way to block VEGF, the growth of new blood vessels could be prevented and the cancer cells could be starved to death.

There is abundant evidence that VEGF is involved in the growth of new blood vessels including those in the wet form of AMD. In a large randomized controlled trial, patients were randomized to receive Macugen® or to a sham treatment that mimicked an injection since Macugen® is injected into the eye like Kenalog®. The results of the trial showed that Macugen® reduced the rate of vision loss in patients with wet AMD compared to patients who received the sham injection. After one year, 70 percent of the AMD patients who received Macugen® had lost fewer than three lines of vision, compared to 55 percent of patients who didn't receive the drug. The injections of the drug were continued for a second year. After two years, on average, the treated patients lost a little less than two lines of vision, whereas the untreated patients lost just over three lines.

The advantage of Macugen® is that it works for all kinds of choroidal neovascularization including the occult type (the slow filling and leaking kind) which didn't respond well to PDT. It is also effective for neovascular membranes that are too large to treat with PDT. The disadvantage is that Macugen® must be injected into the eyeball every six weeks. This brings up the risk of endophthalmitis, an infection in the eye which can be quite serious. About one percent of the patients in this study developed endophthalmitis, but this risk decreased in more recent studies when the doctors took extra special care to make sure that the injection site was free of bacteria. There also appear to be no systemic side-effects from the drug. Patients are often reluctant, however, to return to the doctor every six weeks to have a needle stuck into their eye, even though with proper anesthesia, the injection is only mildly painful at worst. Patients who had Macugen® every six weeks for two years did slightly better than those who had it only for one year. After a year, your doctor can examine your eye and see if you need the injections for a full two years or whether the blood vessels look inactive and you may be able to discontinue the treatments.

Macugen® and Visudyne® both work in the sense that they lower the risk of vision loss to less than what it would be if the patients received no treatment. But, unfortunately, patients with the wet form of AMD still usually lose vision – they just don't lose it as fast as they would without treatment. These two treatments are definite advances but as you can see, they are far from perfect. We need better treatments that stabilize or even bring back vision lost to wet AMD.

Promising Treatments that have not yet been approved in the United States as of February 2006

Lucentis®

Lucentis® is the marketing name given by Genentech, Inc, to ranibizumab, an antibody which binds to vascular endothelial growth factor (VEGF). Lucentis® inhibits all forms of vascular endothelial growth factor. The MARINA Study (an acronym for the Minimally classic/occult trial of the Anti-VEGF antibody Ranibizumab In the treatment of Neovascular AMD) was a large randomized controlled trial. The MARINA study showed that injecting Lucentis® into the eye had much better results than any other treatment for wet AMD. In the study, patients with occult neovascular membranes were randomized to a sham injection or to two different doses of Lucentis® injected into the eye monthly. At twelve months, the treated group had gained about a line and a half of vision compared to a loss of two lines of vision in the control group. This is more than a three line difference in visual acuity between the control and treated groups. Forty percent of treated patients had 20/40 vision after twelve months, which is driving vision in most states. This is the first treatment that has resulted in vision improvement in the wet form of AMD. In this study, less than one percent of patients developed severe sterile inflammation or infectious endophthalmitis. More patients developed mild inflammation in the eye, but this complication seems to have been mostly solved by using a new formulation of the product. Genentech recently announced the excellent results with Lucentis®) held up for two years of follow-up in this study.

The FOCUS Study (the acronym for RhuFab V2 Ocular Treatment Combining the Use of Visudyne™ to Evaluate Safety) was a randomized controlled trial that compared treatment with Visudyne® alone to treatment with Visudyne® along with injections of Lucentis®. The combination group (Visudyne® with injections of Lucentis®) did much better than the Visudyne® only group. The vision results were similar to those found in the treated participants in the MARINA study, in which Lucentis® was used alone without Visudyne®. Therefore, it is unclear whether the addition of Visudyne® improves vision more than Lucentis® alone. The addition of Visudyne® may, however, cause the blood vessels to disappear more quickly and thus reduce the total number of Lucentis® injections in the long run. Many patients had severe inflammation in their eyes when Lucentis® was injected during the same visit as the Visudyne® treatment. This problem of inflammation was almost completely eliminated when Lucentis® was given a week after the Visudyne® treatment and also when a new formula of Lucentis® was used.

ANCHOR is an acronym for "ANti-VEGF Antibody for the Treatment of Predominantly Classic CHORoidal Neovascularization in AMD." ANCHOR was another study that tested Lucentis® against Visudyne®. Patients in the ANCHOR study however, had the type of neovascularization which fills quickly with fluorescein dye and leaks a lot (classic neovascularization), in distinction to the patients in the MARINA study who had neovascularization which fills slowly and leaks less (occult neovascularization). The results of the ANCHOR study showed that Lucentis® was much more effective than Visudyne® at preventing visual loss at one year. That means that Lucentis® prevents vision loss in all types of neovascularization in AMD.

Lucentis® appears to be a more effective treatment than either Visudyne® or Macugen® but it's not yet approved by the FDA. The FDA has granted fast-track status for this drug which means that they will decide whether or not to approve it by the end of June 2006. The only worrisome problem is that, in some of the studies, the patients who received Lucentis® had a slightly greater risk of a heart attack than the control patients. At this point we don't know whether this is a real difference or not.

Avastin®

Avastin®, whose generic name is bevacizumab, is a large antibody that inhibits VEGF. Lucentis® was made by Genentech by cleaving the active portion off of the larger Avastin® molecule. Genentech did this because they thought that the Avastin® molecule was too large to cross the retina and to reach the underlying neovascularization in patients with AMD. Avastin® is FDA approved to treat metatastic colon cancer, for which it is given intravenously.

Avastin® has been given intravenously by a few eye doctors and the preliminary results show that it's a very effective treatment for the abnormal vessels in AMD. The main problem with this treatment is that intravenous Avastin® inhibits VEGF all over the body and therefore has severe side-effects. Most patients who are given

Avastin® develop hypertension which can be severe but is usually treatable. The worst problem, though, is that the drug increases the risk of strokes and heart attacks, some of which were fatal, in people who had the treatment in the clinical trial. The risk of either a stroke or heart attack was each about 2% or a four percent total risk of developing either one of them.

Eye doctors recognized that the results with Lucentis® were better than with other treatments and decided to determine if Avastin® had any effect when it was injected into the eye. They injected very small amounts and the choroidal neovascularization dried up and became inactive. The huge advantage of injecting Avastin® into the eye, as opposed to injecting it into the person's whole system, is that it can be used in much smaller amounts that are only about one three hundredths as large as when used intravenously. Also, since it is confined to the eye and not given intravenously, it shouldn't cause severe side-effects like hypertension or strokes. On the other hand, Genentech took additional manufacturing steps to make sure that Lucentis® would work well in the eye whereas they didn't take these steps with Avastin®. For now though, intraocular injections of Avastin® appear to be safe and effective.

Anecortave Acetate – Retaane®

This is a steroid type drug which inhibits the growth of new blood vessels. It's injected next to the eyeball by making a small incision in the outer coverings of the eye and then inserting a thin tube called a cannula. The drug is slowly injected through the cannula so that it lies next to the surface of the eyeball. The advantage of the drug is that no injection is made into the eyeball itself so there is no risk of endophthalmitis (an infection inside the eye). The other advantage is that it lasts for six months, at which time another injection can be given if necessary.

In a randomized controlled trial, 79 percent of patients who got Retaane® compared to 53 percent of those who received a placebo avoided losing three or more lines of vision. This means that Retaane® reduced the risk of moderate vision loss. The trial was criticized because only 60 percent of patients completed twelve months of follow-up. Usually a high rate of people who drop out of a trial is a warning flag that perhaps the results of the trial cannot be trusted. In this case, however, it can be explained by the fact that the sponsoring company (Alcon) initially intended the trial to last only six months. By the time they decided to extend the study, a number of the patients had already been "closed out," which means they had completed the six months of follow-up and had left the study.

Another trial showed that Retaane® was better than no treatment over a twenty-four month period. A final trial compared Retaane® to treatment with Visudyne® over a twelve-month period. The initial interpretation of the results showed that the two treatments were about equal. In some patients, however, a portion of the drug leaked out into the tears during the injections. When the patients who leaked were eliminated from the analysis, Retaane® appeared to be slightly better than Visudyne®. The FDA has sent Alcon an "approvable" letter, which means that if the company is able to fulfill a few more requirements, the FDA will approve Retaane® for use in patients with AMD. The drug has been approved for use in Australia.

Retaane® will be an attractive option for patients because the injection has to be given only every six months. The medicine is also placed around the eye rather than into it, which eliminates the risk of endophthalmitis. Retaane® is also being tested in another trial (described below) to see whether it can prevent neovascularization from developing in the first place. Retaane® may also be useful as part of a combination treatment. For instance, Lucentis® or Visudyne® could be given first and then Retaane® to prevent the new blood vessels from coming back. This strategy might reduce the number of treatments needed to control the blood vessels.

Treatments aimed at preventing neovascularization in AMD

Even with these new and better treatments for the wet form of AMD, many patients will still lose vision due to scarring beneath the retina. The best treatment would be to prevent the abnormal blood vessels from growing under the retina in the first place. Eye doctors have observed that drusen often disappeared after thermal laser treatment for choroidal neovascularization. That observation led to the idea that maybe very light laser could be given to stimulate the disappearance of the drusen, which in turn might lower the risk of atrophy and neovascularization. The Complications of AMD Trial, or CAPT, is currently testing whether very light laser treatment to the macula reduces the future risk of neovascularization or vision loss. The study has recruited over 1000 patients with AMD who have drusen in both eyes. One of the eyes was randomly chosen to receive a treatment of very light laser burns while the other eye was untreated serving as the control.

Early results from the CAPT and other studies showed that drusen were reduced or even eliminated in many of the eyes that received the laser treatment. The disappearance of drusen may or may not be a good thing, and the study hasn't announced whether the risk of vision loss was lowered or increased in the eyes that received laser. Many of these patients have been followed for five years and the results should be announced in the fall of 2006.

The Prophylactic Treatment of AMD (PTAMD) trial was very similar to the CAPT but used a different laser to treat eyes with drusen. The investigators recently announced that the laser treatment did not reduce the risk of wet AMD nor did it reduce the risk of visual loss. A study from the United Kingdom showed that prophylactic laser hastened the development of wet AMD in the fellow eyes of patients who already had wet AMD in the other eye. Therefore we don't recommend prophylactic laser treatment for drusen at this time.

Another trial aimed at trying to prevent neovascularization is called the Anecortave Acetate Risk Reduction Trial, or AART. Here, anecortave acetate, or Retaane®, is used to try to prevent neovascularization from developing. Patients who have had neovascularization in one eye have about a five to ten percent risk per year of developing abnormal blood vessels in the second eye. The advantage of anecortave acetate, or Retaane®, is that it appears to be very safe and, as we said, involves only one injection around the outside of the eye every six months. The drug appears to inhibit the very early phases of new blood vessel growth, so it may be effective at preventing new blood vessels from starting up in the first place. Over 2500 patients who have had neovascularization in only one eye have been recruited and divided into treatment and control groups, to study whether Retaane® reduces or prevents neovascularization in their second eye. Hopefully, this trial will tell us in a few years whether the injections of Retaane® were helpul If so, AMD patients, especially those who have suffered vision loss in the first eye, may be well advised to get injections of Retaane® twice a year.

Treatments that don't work or are not as good

There are a number of treatments which have been found to be ineffective. These treatments are presented in Insert A at the end of this chapter to keep them clearly separated from the treatments which do work.

What you should do today if you have neovascular, or wet, AMD

The most important thing to know is that any time you develop blurred or distorted vision, you should see an eye doctor right away. After the eye doctor examines your eyes and takes photographs, he or she should be able to explain clearly what is wrong with your eyes. If your doctor cannot explain clearly what is going on, you should ask for a referral. If the eye doctor says you have neovascular, or wet, AMD, it is fair for you to ask whether he or she treats a lot of patients with AMD. Occasionally it may be difficult even for the best eye doctor to be certain whether you have neovascularization. This usually occurs in very early cases of the wet form of AMD. In these cases, the doctor should make arrangements to follow you closely, maybe at intervals of a month or two, as well as tell you to report promptly if your symptoms worsen between visits. He should also give you an Amsler grid so you can check your vision at home.

Remember, if you have any doubt about what your doctor is telling you, you should ask for a referral. The doctor should readily comply. If he doesn't, you can look in the phone book for a doctor who specializes in retinal disease or contact the American Academy of Ophthalmology (see Appendix 6-5 at the end of Chapter Six).

Most patients with the wet form of AMD should have prompt treatment. The currently approved treatments for the wet form of

AMD are thermal laser, Visudyne®, and Macugen®. Visudyne®, and Macugen® result in about a one to two line vision loss over two years, which is better than what happens when there is no treatment. This one or two line loss of vision is the average, so some patients gain vision whereas others lose more than two lines on the chart. Visudyne® seems to work better in combination with an intraocular injection of Kenalog® over the first year but the advantage of adding the Kenalog® may fade after the first year.

Treatment with Lucentis® results in better vision than treatment with PDT, Macugen®, or Retaane® but Lucentis® is not yet FDA approved. Many eye doctors are injecting Avastin® into the eye which seems to have similar results to Lucentis®. Lucentis® and/or Avastin® will probably be the best form of treatment in the near future.

The FDA will probably approve Retaane® but its main role may be to prevent neovascularization from developing in the first place or used in combination treatments.

The Best Treatment for You

How can you tell if you're getting the treatment that's best for you? This is difficult, because even eye doctors can't always tell which eyes will do best with a given treatment. If you're responding to a treatment, however, your vision should be staying about the same or improving. If your vision is worsening, you should see your doctor again. You should also ask your doctor to examine your retina carefully after the first Visudyne® or after the first few Macugen® injections. A good sign is that the fluid beneath the retina is going away and the blood vessels look less active. A bad sign is the opposite; namely, that the blood vessels are enlarging or that the fluid within and under the retina has not gone away or has even increased.

Optical Coherence Tomography, or OCT, results in a cross-section image of the retina, which can help your doctor determine whether a treatment is working. OCT is a quick and painless procedure analogous to having photographs taken of your eye. OCT shows whether the fluid in or under the retina has changed after treatment. The eye doctor can compare the OCT with previous images to see whether you're improving or getting worse. For instance, if the fluid is gone after six weeks, this is a good sign that means the treatment is probably working. If the fluid is still present or worse on the OCT, the doctor should consider using another type of treatment before permanent scarring develops.

Treatment of Neovascularization over the next Few Years

I've said that treatment with Lucentis® results in a gain of one to two lines of vision over one year. Remember though, that patients with AMD usually lose vision from neovascularization before the treatment is given. For instance, a patient with AMD may have 20/25 vision before the neovascularization develops. Then, when the new blood vessels grow and start to leak, the vision drops to 20/100. Treatment with Lucentis® brings the vision back to 20/80 or even 20/60, but that is still a far cry from the original vision of 20/25. There are many new drugs being tested that may be better than Lucentis®. But the best treatment will be to prevent the neovascularization from ever growing in the first place. It's important to follow the dietary and lifestyle guidelines listed in the earlier chapters of this book to reduce your risk of neovascularization.

As we mentioned, Retanne® is being tested in a large trial to see if it can reduce the risk of developing neovascularization in the second eye of patients with wet AMD in the first eye. Hopefully there will be other drugs that will have this effect. It would be ideal if an oral medication could prevent neovascularization.

We also need a treatment for neovascularization that doesn't involve an injection into the eye which is risky. Or at least one in which an injection has to be given infrequently, like once a year. Macugen® and Lucentis® inhibit VEGF but only when they are still present in the eye. What happens when the doctor stops giving injections? It appears that, at least in some patients, the neovascularization starts to come back after the injections are stopped. Neither doctors nor patients want a treatment that means injections have to be given into the eye for the rest of the patient's life.

Possible answers to this problem would be to develop a depot form of the drug which would be slowly released over a long time in the eye thus reducing the number of injections. Another answer might be to combine therapies. For instance, inject Lucentis® to control the neovascularization but also give some Retaane® around the eye to prevent it from coming back at least for the next six months. Or combine Lucentis® with a light Visudyne® treatment.

The progress in the treatment of neovascular AMD is rapid. Every year, we should have better and less risky treatments. For the latest on treatments, you can look on the internet especially on www.medrounds.org/amd/. This is the website of a blog where I discuss the latest in AMD research and treatment.

Table
Current Treatments for Neovascular, or Wet, AMD

I.   Thermal laser – the burning type of laser. Best for neovascularization that doesn't extend beneath the center of the macula.

II.   PDT (Visudyne®) – low intensity (non-burning) laser given to blood vessels after infusion of verteporfin. Best for classic and small blood vessels. Given every three months, usually three or four times.

III.   Macugen® – injected into the eye every six weeks for up to two years. Is effective for any type of neovascular membrane.

IV.   Retaane® – injected outside the eye every six months. Good for any type of neovascular membrane. Not yet approved by FDA but is approved in Australia.

V.   Lucentis® – injected into the eye every four weeks. Only treatment to result in vision improvement. Not yet approved by FDA.

VI.   Avastin® – the larger molecule from which Lucentis® was made. Appears to control wet AMD when injected intraocularly.

VII.   Kenalog® – a corticosteroid injected into the eye usually after Visudyne®. Often has to be given just once or twice.

Insert A
Treatments no longer used for the Wet Form of AMD

Submacular Surgery

The concept of this treatment is simple. A surgeon goes inside your eye, makes a tiny hole in the peripheral part of your macula, passes fine forceps beneath the retina, and removes the abnormal blood vessels. A large randomized trial called the Submacular Surgical Trials compared this surgical treatment to no treatment and basically found no difference in the outcome. The problem seems to be that the abnormal blood vessels are entwined with the normal cells of the retina, especially in the retinal pigment epithelium, and therefore these normal cells are removed along with the blood vessels. This leaves a bare area in the outer retina and RPE which no longer sees. Surgery for neovascular membranes is now seldom recommended by eye doctors.

Some patients with wet AMD develop large hemorrhages beneath the macula. Another one of the Submacular Surgical Trials tested whether removal of this blood surgically was better than observation alone. This surgery didn't increase the chance of improved or stable vision. The surgical group did have a lower risk of severe vision loss (21 percent) compared to the observation group (36 percent). A retinal detachment developed, however, in 16 percent of the eyes which received surgery.

In general there are better treatments now for wet AMD, and submacular surgery is seldom used except perhaps to remove large clots of blood from beneath the macula.

Limited Macular Translocation

This is also a surgical treatment for neovascular AMD. Here, the retina is detached on purpose. Sutures are placed in the outer wall of the eye on the side of the macula to shorten that part of the eye. Then a gas bubble is used to push the retina down toward the bottom of the eye and away from the underlying neovascular membrane in the center of the macula. The abnormal vessels can be removed during surgery or the vessels can be treated after the surgery with laser or PDT. The idea is that early in AMD, the inner retina, including the cone cells, is often fairly intact, and if you could move the macula a little so it lies over a more normal area of RPE, the sight would improve. The surgery works miraculously in a minority of patients, who have an excellent return of vision.

However, the procedure has largely been abandoned for the following reasons:

1. The retina can be moved far enough away from the abnormal vessels only about fifty percent of the time.
2. The blood vessels can recur in the new location.
3. There are possible side-effects from the surgery such as double or tilted vision.
4. A recent study showed that the results of the procedure were no better than with Visudyne® which of course, is much easier.
5. There are now better treatment options for neovascular AMD.

Macular Translocation with 360-Degree Retinotomy

This surgery was developed because the limited macular translocation surgery often didn't move the macula far enough away from the neovascular membrane to improve the patient's sight. In this procedure, the retina is cut loose from its attachment in the periphery and then the entire retina is rotated into a new position. Because the entire retina is loose from its moorings, the macula can be rotated far away from the neovascular vessels. Laser is applied to the retina and then the eye is filled with silicone oil to hold the retina in the new position. A few months later, the silicone is removed and eye muscle surgery is performed to eliminate the tilted image caused by the macula being in a new position. As you can imagine, this is very big surgery for the eye, but, amazingly, a minority of eyes ended up with very good vision.

The surgery is seldom performed anymore since it is so involved; has a high risk of complications, mainly recurrent retinal detachment; and only a few eyes ended up with better vision than can be obtained with less invasive treatments.

Transpupillary Thermal Therapy

Conventional thermal laser involves the use of a high-energy spot of light that is absorbed mainly by pigment in the eye and converted to a burn, which destroys the abnormal blood vessels. Transpupillary thermal therapy uses an infrared laser to gently heat the neovascular vessels which causes the cells in the membrane to gradually die. It was an attractive treatment because it was similar to PDT but without the dye and was therefore quick and easy. The initial studies showed that in some patients, TTT stopped the blood vessels from leaking. Unfortunately, later larger studies, including a randomized controlled trial, showed that TTT was no better than no treatment. A subgroup analysis showed that eyes with poor vision to start with did slightly better with TTT than with no treatment. Overall, however, TTT is not as good as the new treatments and has largely been abandoned.

Radiation

Radiation affects cells that are growing and dividing more than cells that are stable. That's why it's used for cancers, because it will cause more damage to the growing tumor cells than to the normal cells. This was the same theory behind using radiation for the new and proliferating neovascular vessels in AMD. The first few reports on small numbers of patients were encouraging. The larger and better studies that followed, however, showed that radiation was of no benefit in AMD.

Magnets and Electroshock Therapy

There are advertisements touting either magnetic stimulation or electric shock to the macula as a treatment for AMD. The advertisements claim that the treatments cause a revitalization of cells in the macula. These advertisements come with testimonials from grateful patients. The testimonials may seem convincing, but remember that AMD is a variable disease and some patients can improve no matter what. There is also a large placebo effect, in that patients really want to get better, especially after they've spent a lot of money for magnets or an electric shocking device. There have been no articles in scientific journals which have shown a treatment benefit from either of these therapies. I have never seen a patient who has benefited either. The websites selling these devices contain misleading information. It is very difficult to prove that a given treatment does not work except through a large, expensive clinical trial and no trials have been conducted on these treatments, but there is no scientific reason why these treatments should be effective. I know of no expert in the field of macular degeneration who believes that magnets or electric shocks have any benefit in AMD, and I don't recommend them to you.

Insert B
Rheophoresis

Rheophoresis is a procedure that is currently undergoing clinical trials for the treatment of dry AMD. The procedure is analogous to renal dialysis in patients with kidney failure. It involves passing a patient's blood through a machine with filters. The filters in the machine remove high-molecule proteins like cholesterol, and proteins involved in blood clotting, such as fibrinogen and Von Willebrand factor. These substances have been found in Bruch's membrane through which nutrients have to pass on their way from the choriocapillaris to the RPE and cone cells. The theory is that these large-protein molecules might clog the flow of nutrients through Bruch's membrane and incite inflammation, so getting rid of the molecules makes sense in terms of helping people with dry AMD.

One of the problems with this theory is that studies have shown that these large proteins re-accumulate in the blood three or four days after the treatment. But advocates of the procedure say that it may take much longer for the proteins and lipids to re-accumulate in Bruch's membrane. Skeptics say that these large molecules are bound tightly in Bruch's membrane so they would never be removed by the treatment in the first place.

The treatment is expensive and time-consuming and has to be repeated eight times over ten weeks. It's hard to believe that such a temporary procedure would alter a lifetime of bad genes or health habits. Yet two preliminary studies, involving thirty and forty patients respectively, have shown positive results. The results of these studies prompted a larger trial, The Multicenter Investigation of Rheophoresis for AMD (MIRA-1). This trial appears to be well designed with controls. The patients are randomized so that two-thirds of them receive the eight rheophoresis treatments over a ten-week period while one-third of the patients receive a sham treatment. In 2002, the MIRA-1 Study Group announced its one-year results on forty-three patients. On average, the twenty-eight patients who received rheophoresis had 1.6 lines of better visual acuity than the fifteen patients in the placebo group. If these results hold, this could be a new treatment for dry macular degeneration that actually improves vision. The treatment may also lower the risk of developing the wet form of AMD by reducing inflammatory substances in the blood and leeching fats out of Bruch's membrane.

Curiously, however, the results from the same forty-three patients were published again in 2005. The company sponsoring the trial said that the delay of three years was caused by a lack of funding but that now 150 patients had been recruited and more data, according to the sponsors of the trial, will be released early in 2006. The previous publications stated that the data collected by the study was being analyzed by third parties who are not connected with the National Eye Institute or any academic institution. Obviously, a positive result would have huge financial implications for the few companies who provide the equipment for this procedure and these companies are the ones analyzing the data. I will certainly keep an open mind and await the results of the larger study, but the procedures used to analyze the data seem a bit dicey. I would not recommend this treatment at this point because it remains unproven, very expensive, and mildly painful because of the large needles placed in arm veins.

References – Chapter Five

The Anecortave Acetate Clinical Study Group. Anecortave acetate as monotherapy for the treatment of subfoveal lesions in patients with exudative age-related macular degeneration (AMD): interim (month 6) analysis of clinical safety and efficacy. Retina 2003; 23: 14-23.

The Anecortave Acetate Clinical Study Group. Anecortave acetate as monotherapy for treatment of subfoveal neovascularization in age-related macular degeneration: twelve-month clinical outcomes. Ophthalmology 2003; 110: 2372-2385.

The Anecortave Acetate Clinical Study Group. Anecortave acetate as monotherapy for treatment of subfoveal neovascularization in age-related macular degeneration: twelve-month clinical outcomes. Ophthalmology 2003; 110: 2372-2385.

The Eyetech Study Group. Preclinical and phase 1A clinical evaluation of an anti-VEGF pegylated aptamer (EYE001) for the treatment of exudate age-related macular degeneration. Retina 2002; 22: 143-152.

Ferris FL III. A new treatment for ocular neovascularization. N Engl J Med 2004; 351: 2863-2865.

Gragoudas ES, Adamis AP, Cunningham ET Jr, Feinsod M, Guyer DR, for the VEGF Inhibition Study in Ocular Neovascularization Clinical Trial Group. Pegaptanib for neovascular age-related macular degeneration. N Engl J Med 2004; 351: 2805-2816.

Jaakkola A, Heikkonen J, Tommila P, Laatikainen L, Immonen I. Strontium plaque brachytherapy for exudative age-related macular degeneration: three-year results of a randomized study. Ophthalmology 2005; 112: 567-573.

Jonas JB, Spandau UH, Harder B, Vossmerbaeumer U, Kamppeter BA. Intereye difference in exudative age-related macular degeneration with minimally classic or occult subfoveal neovascularization after unilateral intravitreal injection of triamcinolone acetonide. Am J Ophthalmol 2005; 139: 1073-1079).

Klein R, Klein BEK, Knudtson MD, Wong TY, Shankar A, Tsai MY. Systemic markers of inflammation, endothelial dysfunction, and age-related maculopathy. Am J Ophthalmol 2005; 140: 35-44.

Michels S, Rosenfeld PJ, Puliafito CA, Marcus EN, Venkatraman AS. Systemic bevacizumab (Avastin) therapy for neovascular age-related macular degeneration: twelve-week results of an uncontrolled open-label clinical study. Ophthalmology 2005; 112: 1035-1047.

Miller JW, Lane AM. Discussion: Anecortave acetate as monotherapy for treatment of subfoveal neovascularization in age-related macular degeneration: twelve-month clinical outcomes. Ophthalmology 2003; 110: 2384-2385.

The Multicenter Investigation of Rheopheresis for AMD (MIRA-1) Study Group, Pulido JS. Multicenter prospective, randomized, double-masked, placebo-controlled study of rheopheresis to treat nonexudative age-related macular degeneration: interim analysis. Trans Am Ophthalmol Soc 2002; 100: 85-108.

Pieramici DJ, de Juan E Jr, Fujii GY, et al. Limited inferior macular translocation for the treatment of subfoveal choroidal neovascularization secondary to age-related macular degeneration. Am J Ophthalmol 2000; 130: 419-428.

Pulido JS, Sanders D, Klingel R. Rheopheresis for age-related macular degeneration: clinical results and putative mechanism of action. Can J Ophthalmol 2005; 40: 332-340.

Pulido J, Sanders D, Winters JL, Klingel R. Clinical outcomes and mechanism of action for rheopheresis treatment of age-related macular degeneration (AMD). J Clin Apher 2005 Oct;20(3):185-94.

Rechtman E, Danis RP, Pratt LM, Harris A. Intravitreal triamcinolone with photodynamic therapy for subfoveal choroidal neovascularization in age related macular degeneration. Br J Ophthalmol 2004; 88: 344-347.

Spaide RF, Slakter J, Yannuzzi LA, Sorenson J, Freund KB. Large spot transpupillary thermotherapy for occult choroidal neovascularization. Arch Ophthalmol 2005; 123: 1272-1273.

Spaide RF, Sorenson J, Maranan L. Photodynamic therapy with verteporfin combined with intravitreal injection of triamcinolone acetonide for choroidal neovascularization. Ophthalmology 2005; 112: 301-304.

Submacular Surgery Trials (SST) Research Group. Surgery for hemorrhagic choroidal neovascular lesions of age-related macular degeneration: ophthalmic findings: SST Report No. 13. Ophthalmology 2004; 111: 1993-2006.

Submacular Surgery Trials (SST) Research Group. Surgery for subfoveal choroidal neovascularization in age-related macular degeneration: ophthalmic findings: SST Report No. 11. Ophthalmology 2004; 111: 1967-1980.

Treatment of Age-Related Macular Degeneration With Photodynamic Therapy and Verteporfin in Photodynamic Therapy Study Goups. Effect of lesion size, visual acuity, and lesion composition on visual acuity change with and without verteporfin therapy for choroidal neovascularization secondary to age-related macular degeneration: TAP and VIP Report No. 1. Am J Ophthalmol 2003; 136: 407-418.

Treatment of Age-related Macular Degeneration With Photodynamic Therapy (TAP) Study Group. Photodynamic therapy of subfoveal choroidal neovascularization in age-related macular degeneration with verteporfin: one-year results of 2 randomized clinical trials – TAP Report 1. Arch Ophthalmol 1999; 117: 1329-1345.

Treatment of Age-Related Macular Degeneration With Photodynamic Therapy (TAP) Study Group. Photodynamic therapy of subfoveal choroidal neovascularization in age-related macular degeneration with verteporfin: two-year results of 2 randomized clinical trials – TAP Report 2. Arch Ophthalmol 2001; 119: 198-207.

Treatment of Age-Related Macular Degeneration With Photodynamic Therapy (TAP) Study Group. Verteporfin therapy for subfoveal choroidal neovascularization in age-related macular degeneration: four-year results of an open-label extension of 2 randomized clinical trials: TAP Report No. 7. Arch Ophthalmol 2005; 123: 1283-1285.

Treatment of Age-Related Macular Degeneration With Photodynamic Therapy (TAP) Study Group. Verteporfin therapy for subfoveal choroidal neovascularization in age-related macular degeneration: three-year results of an open-label extension of 2 randomized clinical trials – TAP Report No. 5. Arch Ophthalmol 2002; 120: 1307-1314

van Wijngaarden P, Coster DJ, Williams KA. Inhibitors of ocular neovascularization: promises and potential problems. JAMA 2005; 293: 1509-1512.

Verteporfin in Photodynamic Therapy Study Group. Verteporfin therapy of subfoveal choroidal neovascularization in age-related macular degeneration: two-year results of a randomized clinical trial including lesions with occult with no classic choroidal neovascularization – Verteporfin in Photodynamic Therapy Report 2. Am J Ophthalmol 2001; 131: 541-560.

Verteporfin Roundtable Participants. Guidelines for using verteporfin (Visudyne) in photodynamic therapy for choroidal neovascularization due to age-related macular degeneration and other causes: update. Retina 2005; 25: 119-134.

Visudyne in Minimally Classic Choroidal Neovascularization Study Group. Verteporfin therapy of subfoveal minimally classic choroidal neovascularization in age-related macular degeneration: 2-year results of a randomized clinical trial. Arch Ophthalmol 2005; 123: 448-457.

Chapter Six
Vision Rehabilitation by Mark E. Wilkinson, OD

It is a major blow when someone loses vision from AMD, especially when the second eye is affected. The stages of adjusting to any major loss – including shock, anxiety, denial, mourning, and depression – are well known (see Appendix 6-1). Some people with AMD pass through these stages quickly, whereas others require more time and may need professional help to work through them before they come to acknowledgment, acceptance, and finally adjustment and adaptation. If you have AMD, you may be afraid that you are going blind, but we can reassure you that it is rare for someone with AMD to lose all of their vision. We're also rapidly learning more and more about how you can reduce the chances that you'll get AMD in the first place. And the treatments for AMD are improving, so there's a good chance that you'll retain at least some of your central vision if you already have AMD.

About a third of people with AMD become depressed when they lose vision. No one with AMD can afford to be depressed. If you have AMD, you'll need the energy to watch out for new symptoms and to go to the doctor. You'll need to be able to get talking books, to log on to the computer and obtain the latest information, to call your friends for rides if you can't drive, and to socialize. Depression accompanying vision loss sets up a vicious cycle which may cause you to isolate yourself or even give up. Then things will only get worse.

Because healthcare is now so specialized, your eye doctor may not ask you if you're depressed, and your family doctor may not realize how much vision you've lost. You may slip through the cracks, so to speak, unless you tell them you're depressed. Patients these days have to be their own advocates. It's natural for anyone to mourn a loss of vision, but be sure to tell your doctor if you're experiencing any signs of depression, including feelings of sadness or hopelessness, loss of interest in daily activities, weight loss or gain due to a change in your appetite, a feeling that getting up and moving takes a great effort, feelings of guilt or anxiety without an obvious reason, problems concentrating or making decisions, or thoughts of death or suicide. (See Appendix 6-2 for a full list of the signs of depression.).

There are many effective treatments for depression. They include talk therapy, medication, support groups, education about AMD, low vision aids, modifications to your home to make daily living easier, friends or agencies that provide transportation, talking books, support groups, and social or religious organizations. All of these can be considered treatments that will add up to make you feel better. With renewed energy, you'll be amazed at what you can do. Please remember, though, that the crucial first step is to tell one of your doctors how you feel and that you want help.

Vision Loss from AMD

Age-related macular degeneration damages the central part of the retina but usually leaves the peripheral retina intact. The central retina is used for detailed or fine vision. So if you have AMD, you probably have reduced detail vision, which makes it difficult to recognize faces, read, or see well enough to drive. However, since your peripheral retina is still good, you probably have good peripheral, or side vision, and are thus able to ambulate safely and efficiently. The fact that you can travel independently may puzzle your family members and friends, who may wonder why you can't read or recognize their faces yet are able to walk around without bumping into things. They may also notice that you can often see even small objects on the floor. People with normal sight have more trouble understanding the vision loss that comes with AMD than they do understanding total blindness. They can close their eyes and appreciate what it's like to be totally blind, but it's difficult for them to know what it's like to have the decreased detail vision, yet normal peripheral vision, that comes with AMD.

You may worry that your friends will think you're ignoring or even snubbing them because you can't recognize them as they approach. The simplest solution is just to tell them that you can't recognize them and ask them to identify themselves verbally when they approach you. You could also have them read this book. Once they understand what's going on, you need not worry again. In fact, most of your friends will appreciate the fact that you confided in them and will help by telling you when someone's approaching or give you a hand in unfamiliar or dark surroundings.

Macular degeneration not only results in decreased detail vision, represented by reduced visual acuity on an eye chart, it also results in decreased contrast sensitivity. Poor contrast sensitivity makes the world appear hazy or washed out. It also contributes to the difficulty you may be having judging distances, reading printed material, navigating safely in unfamiliar environments, and recognizing faces.

Vision rehabilitation will help you maximize your remaining vision.

What Is Vision Rehabilitation?

Vision rehabilitation is a process involving a number of steps. A vision rehabilitation specialist (Ophthalmologist, MD/DO, Optometrist, OD) will give you an examination to assess your remaining vision and then tailor his or her treatment to your particular needs. He or she will give you tips about how to maximize your vision to make your daily activities easier. The specialist will usually also prescribe one or more vision aids to help you with either your reading or your distance vision or both.

The first step in this process is to consider whether you need to see a rehabilitation specialist. You may already know the answer to that question, but if you don't, Appendix 6-3 at the end of this chapter provides a useful questionnaire for considering your needs and whether vision rehabilitation can help you meet them. If you answer "yes" to any of the questions in Appendix 6-3, then you'd probably benefit from an appointment with a vision rehabilitation specialist.

Sometimes doctors or patients resist the idea of vision rehabilitation. But think of it this way: If you have a knee replacement operation, you're not just sent home. The orthopedic doctor will send you to a rehabilitation specialist who will give you exercises to improve the mobility and strength of the knee. The rehabilitation after surgery is just as important as the surgery itself. In the same way, if you've experienced a loss of vision from age-related macular degeneration, it's natural for you to be referred for a vision rehabilitation evaluation. This evaluation will determine what combination of devices and training is needed so you can make the most of your remaining vision, achieve a sense of well-being, and enjoy a satisfying level of independence.

Although vision rehabilitation makes perfect sense, your eye doctor may forget to refer you for an evaluation. He or she may tell you that nothing more can be done to improve your vision when what your doctor actually means is that nothing more can be done for you medically or surgically. You might therefore have to specifically ask him or her for a referral to a vision rehabilitation specialist.

Even if you have only slightly impaired vision, a referral may be helpful. There is no required amount of visual acuity or visual field loss for someone to be referred for vision rehabilitation, and often people with less vision loss are helped the most. In addition, it may be easier to learn how to use various vision aids when you still have pretty good vision. Therefore, we would recommend that you ask for an appointment with a vision rehabilitation specialist anytime you're having problems or if your doctor tells you it's likely that you'll lose more vision in the future.

Comprehensive Care for AMD

If you have AMD, you should be sure that you get the following three phases of treatment:

1. You should have an initial evaluation by an eye doctor who provides a diagnosis and medical treatment, or a referral for treatment. An eye doctor experienced in AMD should continue to follow and treat you if necessary, probably for the rest of your life.

2. If you're having problems with your vision or your eye doctor thinks there's a chance that you'll lose more vision, you should be evaluated by a vision rehabilitation specialist. The specialist will evaluate your vision, prescribe vision aids, and suggest lifestyle modifications to help you with your problems.

3. You need to be trained in how to use any vision aids you've been prescribed. You should have periodic follow-up appointments with the vision rehabilitation specialist so he or she can assess your

progress and make sure the problems you were having have been helped, as well as address new problems you may be experiencing.

The Vision Rehabilitation Visit

Vision rehabilitation is goal-directed, meaning it's focused on helping you perform specific problematic tasks. Usually during a visit to a vision rehabilitation specialist, the specialist or his or her helper takes a comprehensive history of what has happened to your eyes. He or she will ask what problems you're having with your vision and ask specifically whether you're having problems with your activities of daily living, your ability to travel independently, or your ability to carry on your favorite recreational or social activities.

The specialist will test your vision using special charts and evaluate the benefits of devices designed for patients who have lost vision. He or she will encourage you to do as well as you can, but you'll find that these tests are not taxing or threatening. The specialist will then prescribe a vision aid to help you with your problem.

Vision Rehabilitation Options

Vision rehabilitation specialists consider illumination, contrast enhancement and magnification as initial treatment options for enhancing vision. Magnification works by increasing the size of the image on your retina so that enough retinal cells are stimulated to send a detailed image to your brain. This, in turn, allows you to see and identify the object. There are four types of magnification:

1. Relative distance magnification. When you hold something closer to your eye, it appears bigger. So, for example, moving closer to the television will enlarge both the image and the brightness of the screen, making it easier to see the TV. Since it's hard to focus on objects that are very close to your eyes, stronger bifocals or special reading glasses are often prescribed to help you focus on print or an object of interest.

2. Relative size magnification means making the object larger so it can be seen. This concept is used in large print books or notes written by hand in large letters.

3. Angular magnification means making a smaller object look bigger to your eye by using a magnifying lens or a telescope.

4. Electronic magnification uses a camera hooked to a television or computer screen to enlarge an object. The electronic controls also allow you to increase the brightness and contrast of the image on the screen.

Devices Used in Vision Rehabilitation

Stronger Bifocals

The vision specialist will first check your distance vision, usually by putting a trial frame which simulates eyeglasses on your face. The trial frame contains slots that hold lenses and allows the specialist to accurately determine which lenses you see best with for both distance and near vision. The specialist will note the level of your distance and near vision which will give him a strong hint as to what magnification you'll need for near tasks such as reading. Sometimes the only thing needed for reading is a stronger bifocal lens. In general, the specialist will give you the least amount of lens power that is needed for you to see clearly. Lower-powered lenses have a longer focal or working distance than higher-powered lenses, which means you can hold reading material farther away, at a more comfortable position.

Spectacle Magnifiers

If stronger bifocals don't give you enough magnification to read or see close objects, the specialist may recommend a spectacle magnifier. These are stronger lenses mounted in an eyeglass frame. They are basically like very strong bifocals. The advantages of spectacle magnifiers are that they free your hands for other tasks and provide a wider field of vision than other comparable devices. This wider field of view allows you to see a number of words at a time which will increase your reading speed more than other devices of similar power.

One disadvantage of spectacle magnifiers is that they may be tiring because they require you to hold reading material or objects very close to the glasses in order to bring them into focus. Also, people with AMD need a lot of light to see well and it may be difficult to get enough light on the reading material because it must be held so close to these eyeglasses. The short distance also makes it hard to write while looking through the magnifying lenses.

When objects are held close to the eyes, both eyes have to turn inward (toward the nose), in order to see one image; this is called convergence. The eyes often cannot turn in enough to focus on very close objects, including reading material held close while wearing spectacle magnifiers. In lower powers, this problem is alleviated by prisms added to the magnifying lenses. When higher corrections are needed, the rehabilitation specialist will often recommend spectacle magnifiers with only one magnifying lens, usually for the eye with better vision.

Hand and Stand Magnifiers

The vision rehabilitation specialist may recommend that you use a hand magnifier like the ones used by detectives in old movies. Hand magnifiers come in a variety of strengths and designs. One important consideration is that the stronger the magnifier is, the smaller the lens diameter and field of view. If you have a small field of view, you may see only one word or even just a few letters of a word at a time which makes it difficult to read smoothly. An advantage of hand magnifiers is that they can be used to read or look at something from a farther, more ordinary distance than can be done with spectacle-mounted magnifiers. The longer working distance is less tiring and makes it relatively easy to get good light on the object or reading material. Many of the magnifiers have their own source of light built right into them. Hand magnifiers are also familiar and easy to use. They're convenient for spot-reading tasks like reading price tags. They are also inexpensive, portable, and can be used with your regular eyeglasses.

A disadvantage of hand magnifiers is that they must be held at a specific distance. This may make high-powered hand magnifiers almost impossible to use for some people with limited dexterity or tremors, because any little movement is magnified greatly. They also have a smaller field of view, so using them for prolonged reading can be slow and uncomfortable.

Stand magnifiers are high-powered lenses mounted in a frame (usually plastic) with sides or feet that stand on top of reading material. The height of the frame varies with the power of the lens and is set to bring the object into focus. One advantage of stand magnifiers is that they're stable and don't move. They can therefore be used in higher powers or by someone with tremors. You can read at a close to normal distance with a stand magnifier, which reduces fatigue. They also often have built-in light sources.

A disadvantage of stand magnifiers is that they're larger than reading glasses or hand magnifiers, which make them a bit less portable. Stand magnifiers can also be awkward to use on non-flat surfaces, so they wouldn't be as helpful as reading glasses or hand magnifiers for tasks such as reading the labels on cans. The stand can cause a shadow on the text or object unless it has a built-in light. It is impossible to write while using most stand magnifiers.

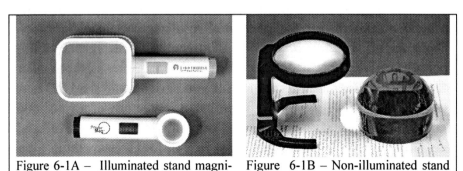

Figure 6-1A – Illuminated stand magnifiers

Figure 6-1B – Non-illuminated stand Magnifiers

Telescopes

Telescopes use a combination of lenses, prisms, and mirrors to magnify objects. A telescope can be handheld up to the eye or mounted on spectacles and can be used with one or both eyes. Some telescopes can be focused like cameras so they're useful for looking at both close and far away objects. That means you can use the same device to read a letter or to see a bird at your feeder.

A disadvantage of telescopes is that they have a small field of view so you may have to search around for the object you want to see. The luminance, or brightness, of viewed objects is reduced with telescopes which can reduce their effectiveness. Telescopes vary in price from less than $100 to several thousand dollars, depending on whether they're handheld or spectacle mounted as well as whether they're for use by one or both eyes.

Implantable Miniaturized Telescope (IMT)

This is a telescope that is placed inside the eye of patients with severe AMD after a cataract is removed. So far ophthalmologists have placed the IMT in the eyes of about 200 individuals. The miniature telescope is being studied as part of a FDA Phase II/III clinical trial which completed enrollment in the fall of 2003. One year after implantation, 90 percent of the individuals who had received this device had gained two or more lines of vision at distance or near. It is unknown how much of this improvement was the result of simply removing the cataract and how much was due to the telescope.

The telescope places a magnified image on the macula which may be useful if there is remaining macular function. Since the image is just on the macula, the peripheral visual field will not be of much use. Often the peripheral vision is the only remaining vision in an eye with severe AMD. The limitation of peripheral vision may make it harder for someone to travel independently or orient themselves. It will be impossible to use both eyes together since the image in one eye will be highly magnified compared to the other eye. It's not known when and if this device will become available for the general public but currently we don't recommend it.

Video Magnification

Video magnification devices use high-resolution cameras hooked up to television or computer screens to magnify objects or written materials which are placed in front of the cameras. These devices are capable of very high magnification. You can literally make one letter in a word fill the entire screen. Video magnifiers also have adjustments and can be set to provide very bright illumination as well as maximal contrast enhancement (see below). You can use both eyes to view the screen and you can place writing materials under the camera. Even at high magnification, the field of view provided by the screen is relatively large and allows for a reasonable reading speed. In other words, you can read fast enough to understand what you're reading. The amount of magnification can be adjusted for different sizes of materials or fluctuations in vision. Since the reading material or object is place under the camera and then left there, video magnifiers are good for people with physical impairments, loss of dexterity, or hand tremors.

A disadvantage of closed circuit television devices is that they're less portable than other devices. However, newer portable devices are now available. Closed-circuit television devices vary in price from several hundred dollars to several thousand dollars. An individualized evaluation in a vision rehabilitation clinic is necessary to determine which of the many types of closed-circuit television devices is best for you. Training is needed to be able to use these devices quickly and efficiently. As with all other devices, some individuals will find closed-circuit television devices hard to use.

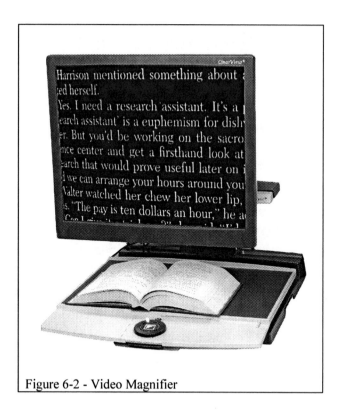

Figure 6-2 - Video Magnifier

Head-Borne Magnifiers

Head-borne video magnification devices allow for distance, intermediate, and near vision enhancement with variable levels of magnification and contrast enhancement. The advantages of head-borne video magnification devices are that they provide variable levels of magnification for near, intermediate, and distance tasks; they provide contrast enhancement; they allow for binocularity (using both eyes at the same time) at high levels of magnification; they make it possible for manipulative tasks to be performed with both hands; their level of magnification can be easily adjusted for different sizes of materials or fluctuations in vision; and they can provide direct input from the television.

The disadvantages of head-borne video magnification devices are that they're somewhat heavy when worn for extended periods of time; they require relatively good head control; they're more expensive than other devices; and they require orientation and training to be used effectively.

Non-optical Devices

Your vision rehabilitation specialist may also recommend non-optical devices such as large-print books, playing cards, or bingo cards. You may want to use bold-ruled white paper and black felt-tip pens to write letters or notes so that they can be read easily. You may also find devices which depend on hearing rather than sight to be helpful such as talking clocks, watches, or calculators.

Reading stands can be adjusted to an optimal height when you're standing or sitting so as to reduce body fatigue from an abnormal posture. You can also get large-print checks or stencil guides with slots in them so that you can keep within the lines when writing checks.

You may find that mini-tape recorders are easier to use than writing out notes or shopping lists. There is also a text-to-speech synthesizer program that can be loaded on your computer. The program allows your computer to read aloud anything on its screen, as well as any files stored on your computer or downloaded from the Internet. Couple the synthesizer with the internet, and you should have ready access to the world.

Special Issues

Glare

If you have AMD, you've probably noticed that you need much brighter light to see well. On the other hand, you may have also noticed that glare bothers you and decreases your vision. This is a conundrum – the need for more light, yet the glare that can be caused by brighter light. Luckily there are certain lenses, called absorptive lenses, which cut glare without cutting much of the light. These lenses are available in a variety of different styles, including ones that slip over or behind your glasses or ones that can simply be put on like regular eyeglasses. These absorptive lenses block ultra-violet light, reduce glare, improve contrast, and may improve visual acuity. In some people, however, they may reduce visual acuity and alter the color of objects. If glare is a problem for you, ask your vision rehabilitation specialist about absorptive lenses.

You can also cut glare with window shades, anti-reflective coatings on spectacles, polarized coatings, and special lighting and light bulbs. Another good tip is to put any reading material on top of a dark, non-reflective mat. That way only the reading material is illuminated. When you go outside, you can control glare by wearing a wide-brimmed hat, visor, or ball cap, all of which reduce extraneous glare coming from the sun or overhead lights.

Illumination

You may find that you see worse at home than you did at the vision rehabilitation evaluation. The problem may be that the lighting in your home isn't bright enough. In their book *Vision and Aging*, Rosenbloom and Morgan state, "Poor lighting in the home is virtually a universal problem."

Strong illumination is the single most important factor in enhancing vision functioning. A low vision clinic found that 1188 lux (the unit of measurement for illumination) is the optimal amount for people with vision impairments, yet the lighting in a normal home averages only 177 lux. The same study showed that more than 90 percent of people with vision impairments showed improvement in near and distance visual acuity when their illumination was improved.

General home lighting does not provide the correct amount of illumination to perform tasks such as reading, writing, and threading a needle. Task lighting is needed to perform these tasks comfortably and efficiently. Task lights should be positioned and adjusted to avoid glare. Try to angle the light to fall over your shoulder on the side of your better eye and then position the reading materials where you can see best. You should experiment with various positions of the light source, the reading material, and your body position to see what's best for you. An adjustable lamp with an incandescent indoor floodlight bulb of 60 to 100 watts will provide good illumination and contrast.

You may find that it's useful to carry a small flashlight with a bright beam to help you walk in dark restaurants or movie theaters. You may also want to carry a magnifying lens with built-in illumination so you can read the menu in dark restaurants.

Contrast

We've already mentioned contrast many times in this chapter. People with AMD have reduced vision as measured on a visual acuity chart, but that doesn't tell the whole story. They also have problems with contrast sensitivity. Contrast vision is the ability to discern one object from another, for instance, to see the coffee cup on the placemat. That's why a person with AMD will be able to read a letter written in black ink on white paper much better than one written in red ink on pink paper. You can make your day-to-day activities in your home much easier by enhancing contrast. For example, white dishes on a dark tablecloth will be much easier for you to see than purple dishes on a blue tablecloth. You may want to shake salt and pepper onto your hand before sprinkling them on your food since they're often hard to see when they come out of shakers.

You may find it helpful to mark often-used settings in some way that will increase their contrast and make them easier to see. For example, settings on the stove or oven, the washer or dryer, and the thermostat for the air conditioner or furnace, can be marked with a thick swipe of bright-colored fabric paint or nail polish. Jars and canned goods can be relabeled using a thick black marker on index cards. After the jars or cans have been used, the old index cards can be used to make shopping lists. You can choose personal hygiene articles with bright containers or caps in order to find them easily in the bathroom. You can also mount a magnifying mirror in the bathroom to help with shaving or applying make-up. If your bathroom wall is dark, choose white towels for contrast. If the walls are light choose darker towels. And make sure there's plenty of light in your closets.

Sight Substitution

In some cases, you may choose to substitute your sense of hearing for your sense of sight. Books and magazines on tape or CD are becoming increasingly available at local libraries or bookstores. The National Library Service for the Blind and Physically Handicapped in the Library of Congress has developed an extensive talking books program. They offer almost every kind of book and magazine and the program provides everything free of charge including playback equipment and shipping costs. The address for this service is given in Appendix 6-5 under "Library of Congress."

You can also try the popular Radio Reading Information Services, which is free for those who are visually impaired. Radio Information Services are regional services that broadcast a variety of local daily and weekly newspapers, magazines, short stories, and best-selling and classic novels to their listeners 24 hour a day, 7 days a week. This service requires a special receiver that is provided free of charge by the service provider in your area. You can contact your state's Department for the Blind/Department for Rehabilitative Services or your local low vision rehabilitation provider to find out how to get signed up for this service. You can also try Disability Radio Worldwide (DRW), which has a variety of offerings for people with impaired sight (see Appendix 6-5 for the website address).

The vast majority of people with macular degeneration retain enough vision to be able to continue doing their daily reading activities with the help of magnification devices. For this reason, Braille instruction is not normally pursued by individuals with macular degeneration. Those who do pursue Braille instruction often find it difficult to get to the level of Braille proficiency where they can read fluently. That being said, Braille can still be beneficial for labeling clothing and other items such as canned goods. As an alternative, you may find it useful to use different ways of marking jars and other containers, such as putting one piece of coarse tape on corn and two pieces on beans, et cetera, or any other scheme that allows you to identify the contents of the container by touch.

Ambulation

If you have severe vision loss due to macular degeneration, you may find it helpful to use a white cane when you walk. A white cane can help you avoid obstacles or holes and also identify yourself as someone with vision loss. If you do opt to use a white cane, you'll need to get proper training in order to use it to its best advantage. Usually an orientation and mobility specialist provides this training and is available through state-sponsored rehabilitation services as well as some hospital-based rehabilitation centers. Occupational and physical therapists can also provide some ambulation training.

When you travel with someone who is normally sighted, it's helpful to use the Human Guide Technique. You should lightly grasp your guide's arm just above his or her elbow. Your guide should walk slowly and steadily and approach curbs, stairs, and doorways squarely and never at an angle. He or she should let you know when to step up or down and should always stay a half-step ahead of you so you can sense when she's stepping up or down even if she forgets to tell you.

Driving with a Vision Impairment

A major concern for people over 65 is the loss of their ability to drive. Appendix 6-4 at the end of this chapter is a driving questionnaire that we give patients in our vision rehabilitation clinic. Even people with normal vision often have some of the problems listed in the questionnaire, so if you answer "yes" to some of the questions it doesn't necessarily mean you should give up driving, however, the questionnaire will give you an idea of how much trouble your vision is causing when you're driving. Most people with AMD have a pretty good idea of whether they're safe to drive or not. The problem is, even if you still feel safe driving, you may not be visually "legal" to drive in your state.

Currently, each state has widely different laws determining who can and cannot have a driver's license. The minimum level of visual acuity allowed for driving ranges from 20/40 to 20/200 in different states. Some states have no visual field restrictions, while others require a minimum visual field that ranges from 40 to 140 degrees. For this reason it is impossible for us to make a general statement about how much vision you need in order to keep your driver's license. You can contact your local driver's license bureau for more information.

There are other factors besides vision which determine whether someone is a safe driver. The biggest factor, in our experience, is the driver's cognitive ability. The biggest threat on the roads is probably a driver with dementia, not one with vision problems.

You may be tempted to continue to drive if you have an unexpired license even though you have lost vision since your last licensing test. This could be dangerous and could cause you to hurt yourself or others. It may also be illegal, since most states require that you report any change in your health, mental condition, or vision which may affect your driving. Failure to report vision loss may also make your car insurance invalid and lay you open to legal problems.

The right solution is to see a vision rehabilitation specialist. The specialist will tell you whether you visually qualify to continue driving, at least on a limited basis. They can also serve as your advocate if you need an eye doctor's statement that you are still visually competent to drive in order to maintain driving privileges. The licensing authorities may ask you to take a "behind the wheel test" with a licensing examiner. Individuals with AMD who successfully pass this test are allowed to continue to drive. Often times, however, the licensing bureau will restrict them to daylight driving only or to driving under a certain speed. This usually works out well because it allows the person to pick out the time and route they use to accomplish their needed tasks.

Agencies and Services

Depending on your vision, you may be able to get free directory assistance through your local phone company. The operator will look up phone numbers for you and even dial the number. To qualify for this, request a form from your phone company which can be signed by your doctor or vision rehabilitation specialist.

Appendix 6-5 at the end of this chapter lists agencies that provide assistance with daily living (ADL) such as ride programs and meals on wheels.

Funding Issues

The cost of optical devices should be, but aren't covered by most insurance policies, including Medicare. However, Medicare and some insurance companies usually do pay at least part of the bill for an appointment to a vision rehabilitation specialist. Many states also fund vision rehabilitation evaluations and devices for select individuals. Funding may also be available from service organizations, such as Lions Clubs. These appointments and devices are important, so we encourage you to do everything possible to try to find the necessary funds. The Lions Clubs have been generous in offering help, but we believe that the state and federal government should fund vision rehabilitation and devices. They're a good value because they allow people with AMD to remain independent and functional for a relatively low cost.

Follow-Up

You'll need instruction to learn how to get the best use of whatever devices your vision rehabilitation specialist prescribes. Most vision rehabilitation specialists or their staff will instruct you on how to use the devices and then give you a free trial period of several weeks. After a few weeks, you should go back to the specialist so he or she can reassess how you're doing and determine whether you need any modification of the device or even whether you need something different. Please keep trying. Just imagine trying to learn how to hit a golf ball after just one lesson. It takes time and effort to learn how to use these devices, but it's worth it.

Other Issues for Someone with Vision Loss

If you have lost vision in both eyes you may have hallucinations. These may be simple hallucination such as streaks of light, or they may be complex hallucinations of objects and people and sometimes even whole scenes that move. The formed hallucinations have been termed the Charles Bonnet Syndrome after the man who described them after talking to his blind grandfather in 1769. Both types of hallucinations are thought to be a "release phenomenon" in the brain, which occur because the brain isn't getting the normal impulses from the eye. You may be concerned by what you're "seeing" or be reluctant to tell your doctor because you fear you may be going crazy or getting senile, but the hallucinations have no medical significance and are common. You should mention them to your doctor mainly so he or she can reassure you. Most people never get to the point where they enjoy their hallucinations but with reassurance they're usually able to ignore them or even laugh when they tell others about what they're "seeing."

Falls are a common cause of injury and even death in many older people. The major causes of falls are hip fractures from osteoporosis or anything that causes reduced blood flow to the brain, including strokes, heart arrhythmias, or low blood pressure. If you're the age when falls are common, you should keep the pathways in your home clear of obstructions. Steps should be clearly marked, even to the point of putting bright orange tape along their edges. Hold onto the rail of the steps. You should also take your time when going from dark rooms into bright light outside or vice versa, in order to give your eyes time to adjust. Try to arrange your bed so you can turn on the lights if you have to get up in the middle of the night. When you get up in the night, turn on the lights and sit on the side of the bed for a minute or two. This will ensure that your eyes have adjusted and your blood pressure will not be too low when you first stand up.

You may notice that your vision varies from day to day or even during the day. This is a common complaint that eye doctors don't fully understand. You might want to pay attention to the conditions when you see best and then try to replicate them. If your vision is worse for more than a day, you should check with your eye doctor. Most people can differentiate between these simple daily fluctuations of vision and a new distortion or blurring of their vision caused by the growth of abnormal blood vessels. When in doubt, call your eye doctor.

Summary

We have tried to keep this chapter upbeat and positive. That doesn't mean, however, that we're minimizing your loss of vision. We know how frustrating it is to lose vision. You should know, though, that using your remaining vision will not worsen your macular degeneration. In fact, using your vision has a positive effect in retraining the brain to interpret images more easily. So please don't give up. Fight. There are specialists to help you with depression. There are many agencies to help you. Comprehensive vision rehabilitation services will help you regain control of your life. Your glass is half full, not half empty, and you can fill it even more by taking advantage of all of the available treatments and vision aids.

Appendix 6-1

Stages of Adjustment to a Loss

1st – Shock
2nd –Anxiety
3rd – Bargaining
4th – Denial
5th – Mourning
6th – Depression
7th – Withdrawal
8th – Internalizing anger
9th – Externalizing anger
10th – Acknowledgment
11th – Acceptance
12th – Adjustment, Adaptation

Appendix 6-2

Are You Depressed?

We recommend that you see your family doctor or a mental health professional if you have had five or more of the following symptoms for more than two weeks, or if any one of these symptoms has interfered with your life.

- You feel sad or cry a lot.
- You feel guilty for no reason.
- You feel that you're no good.
- You've lost your confidence.
- You feel that your life is meaningless
- You believe that nothing good is ever going to happen again.
- You feel negative a lot of the time.
- You have no emotions or feelings.
- You no longer want to do the things you used to enjoy.
- You don't want to be with friends. You want to be left alone.
- You have trouble making decisions.
- You forget things or can't concentrate.
- You get irritated a lot. You lose your temper over little things.
- You don't sleep like you used to. You sleep a lot more. You have trouble falling asleep. Or you wake up early in the morning and can't get back to sleep.
- You have lost your appetite or you now eat a lot more.
- You feel restless and tired most of the time.
- You think about death or feel like you're dying.
- You think about killing yourself.

Do You Need Vision Rehabilitation?

To determine your need for low vision rehabilitation services, please answer the following questions. Because of your vision, are you having trouble with:

1.	Reading regular-size printed materials?	Yes	No
2.	Signing your name on a document?	Yes	No
3.	Making a phone call without operator assistance?	Yes	No
4.	Telling time on a watch or clock?	Yes	No
5.	Managing your personal affairs?	Yes	No
6.	Recognizing people?	Yes	No
7.	Watching TV?	Yes	No
8.	Performing activities of daily living (cooking, sewing, shopping, or personal grooming)?	Yes	No
9.	Driving or being fearful when you drive?	Yes	No
10.	Traveling independently at home or in the community?	Yes	No

How do you feel about your life right now, on a scale of 1 to 10, with one being the worst and ten being the best?

_____

_____

If you answered "Yes" to any of the questions above, or if problems with your vision are decreasing your satisfaction with life, you may benefit from low vision rehabilitation services.

1. Do you have difficulty reading all of the in-
    struments on your car's dashboard clearly and
    rapidly either in daylight, at dusk, on a cloudy
    day, or at night?   Yes   No

2. Do you have difficulty reading road signs in
    time to comfortably react to them either in
    daylight, at dusk, a cloudy day, or at night?   Yes   No

3. Do other cars on the road unexpectedly ap-
    pear to "pop" into and out of your field of
    vision?   Yes   No

4. When driving, do you drive well below the
    speed limit and slower than most cars around
    you either in daylight, at dusk, or at night?   Yes   No

5. When driving, do you have difficulty posi-
    tioning yourself on the road with respect to
    other cars, the lines on a road, curves, side-
    walks, parking spaces, etc., either in daylight,
    at dusk, or at night?   Yes   No

6. When driving, do you find yourself feeling
    confused, stressed, lost and/or disoriented ei-
    ther in daylight, at dusk, or at night?   Yes   No

7. Are your friends or family members worried
    about your driving?   Yes   No

8. Have you had any driving errors or "near
    misses" in the past six months?   Yes   No

9. Do left-hand turns make you nervous?   Yes   No

10. Do you have difficulty turning the steering wheel, or pushing down on the gas pedal or brakes?   Yes   No

11. Do you have trouble looking over your shoulder when backing up?   Yes   No

12. Do people no longer accept rides from you?   Yes   No

13. Do you always remember to wear your seat belt?   Yes   No

14. Is your health (including vision) stable?   Yes   No

15. Has your eye care specialist or vision rehabilitation specialist said you could drive with your condition?   Yes   No

16. Has your general practitioner said you can drive with your condition?   Yes   No

17. Do you want to go through the steps necessary to acquire or retain a low vision driver's license?   Yes   No

Appendix 6-5
Resource List

Organizations that are helpful resources for those with vision impairment:

American Academy of Ophthalmology
P.O. Box 7424
San Francisco, CA 94109-1336
Phone: 415-561-8500

http://www.aao.org/

AAO provides brochures and eye fact sheets on visual impairment and related eye conditions.

American Association of Retired Persons (AARP)
55 ALIVE Driver Safety Program
601 E Street, NW
Washington, DC 20049
Phone: 888-227-7669

www.aarp.org/55alive

Visit the website to find safety driving tips, information on aging and driving, and details about the 55 ALIVE Driver Safety Program – a classroom course for drivers age 50 and older. In this course, participants review driving skills and learn tips to help them drive more safely. Call the toll-free number or visit the website to find a class in your area.

American Automobile Association (AAA)
Foundation for Traffic Safety
607 14th Street NW, Suite 201
Washington, DC 20005
Phone: 800-993-7222

www.aaafoundation.org

Free booklets on traffic safety are available by calling their toll free number or visiting their website.

American Council of the Blind
1155 15th St. NW, Suite 720
Washington, DC 20005
Phone: 800-424-8666

www.acb.org

Membership organization of persons who are blind or visually impaired along with state chapters. Publishes a monthly magazine, "The Braille Forum" in large print, tape, or Braille. Special interest groups include lawyers, teachers, and a variety of others.

American Foundation for the Blind
11 Penn Plaza, Suite300
New York, NY 10001
Phone 800-232-5463

www.afb.org

Serves as a national clearinghouse for information about blindness and referral database. Publishes books, pamphlets, videos, and periodicals about blindness and "Directory of Agencies Serving the Visually Impaired in the U.S."

American Optometric Association
243 North Lindbergh Blvd.
St. Louis, MO 63141-7881
Phone: 800-365-2219

www.aoa.org

The American Optometric Association provides information on macular degeneration and services for individuals with visual impairments. The association can assist in referring individuals to local sources for optometric/low vision services.

Area Agency on Aging (AAA)
Elder Locator: 1-800-677-1116

www.aoa.gov

The local Area Agency on Aging can connect you to services in the area, including ride programs, Meals-on-Wheels, home health services, etc. Call the toll free number or visit the website to find the phone number for your local Area Agency on Aging.

Association for Driver Rehabilitation Specialists (ADED)
1-800-290-2344

www.driver-ed.org or www.aded.net

Call the toll free number or visit the website to find a driver rehabilitation specialist in your area.

Association for Macular Diseases, Inc.
210 East 64th Street
New York, NY 10021
Phone: 212-605-3719

www.macula.org

Promotes education on and research into macular diseases in addition to providing support for affected persons and their families.

Blinded Veterans Association
477 H Street, NW
Washington, DC 20001-2694
Phone: 800-669-7079

www.bva.org

BVA is the only veteran's service organization chartered by the U.S. Congress to represent blinded veterans. BVA Field Reps can help veterans establish claims, attend blind rehabilitation, and regain their rightful place in society. Membership is not required for any service and a national newsletter is available upon request.

Foundation Fighting Blindness
11435 Cronhill Drive
Owings Mills, MD 21117-2220
Phone: 800-683-5555

www.blindness.org

Supports research and provides information on macular degeneration and other degenerative eye diseases.

National Association of Social Workers (NASW)

www.socialworker.org

A social worker can provide counseling to assess social and emotional needs and to assist in locating and coordinating transportation and community services. To find a clinical social worker in your area, search the NASW Register of Clinical Social Workers at their website under Resources.

National Eye Institute (NEI)
2020 Vision Place
Bethesda, MD 20892-3655
Phone: 301-496-5248

www.nei.nih.gov/

One of the United States' National Institutes of Health; the NEI "conducts and supports research that helps prevent and treat eye diseases and other disorders of vision."

Prevent Blindness America (PBA)
211 West Wacker Drive, Suite 1700
Chicago, IL 60606
Phone: 800-331-2020

www.preventblindness.org

PBA is a leading volunteer eye health and safety organization dedicated to fighting blindness and saving sight. PBA works through patient, public and professional, education, community programs and research.

Social Security Administration
6401 Security Blvd.
Baltimore, MD 21235
Phone: 800-772-1213

www.ssa.gov

A resource concerning disability benefits related to legal blindness and other disabilities.

VisionConnection

www.visionconnection.org

Founded by Lighthouse International, VisionConnection is a one-stop, accessible online resource on vision impairment and vision rehabilitation for people who are partially sighted or blind, the professionals who work with them, the families and friends who support them and anyone looking for the latest information on prevention, research and treatment.

WebMD Health

www.webmd.com

An online provider of health information.

Large Print/Taped/Braille Materials

American Federation for the Blind

Customer Service, AFB Press
11 Penn Plaza, Suite 300
New York, NY 10001
800-232-3044

www.afb.org/services.asp

Locates organizations in the United States and Canada that provide services to people who are blind or visually impaired and their families. The Service Center is based on the AFB Directory of Services for Blind and Visually Impaired Persons in the United States and Canada.

American Printing House for the Blind

P. O. Box 6085
Louisville, KY 40206-0085
Phone: 800-223-1839

www.aph.org

APH is the world's largest not-for-profit company devoted solely to create products for visually impaired persons of all ages. APH provides: 1) a variety of products and accessible books, 2) a quick, complete, centralized method of locating materials in accessible media created by agencies and organizations across the nation,

3) custom products of informational materials in accessible formats, 4) free accessible APH catalogs on request.

Aurora Ministries
P. O. Box 621
Bradenton, FL 34206
Phone: 941-748-3031

http://aurora.gospelcom.net

Bible on cassette or CD is available free in 46 languages to persons with print handicaps, low vision, or visual impairments. Complimentary sets are provided for use in resource centers of libraries.

Braille Bible Foundation
PO Box 948307
Maitland, FL 32794-8307
Phone: 800-766-9080 or 407-834-3628
Fax: 407-834-9953

Offers large-print Bible in 16- and 24-point type free to those who are legally blind. Available in Braille form and on tape.

Choice Magazine Listening
85 Channel Drive
Port Washington, NY 11050
Phone: 888-724-6423

www.choicemagazinelistening.org

CML is a free audio anthology available to vision impaired, blind or physically disabled adults from college age and older. The anthology is produced on the special-speed four-track cassette format, playable on the free Library of Congress 4-track cassette player, and provided nationwide. Issues are bi-monthly and provide eight hours of unabridged selected articles, short stories, and poetry. Issues are free to keep and are available to individuals or facilities.

Computer Screen - Vision Enhancement
Look up ways to make your computer more sight-friendly at microsoft.com/enable or apple.com/disability

Disability Radio Worldwide (DRW)

Jean Parker, a disability advocate and radio producer, has a weekly radio show that is currently on the web at www.acbradio.org every Wednesday at 9:30 p.m. EST. After the original broadcast the show will be played every two hours for a 24-hour period.
DRW has other websites www.acbradio.mainstream and www.independentliving.org/radio.

Guideposts Associates, Inc.

39 Seminary Hill Road
Carmel, NY 10512
Phone: 800-932-2145

www.guidepost.org

Monthly interfaith inspirational magazine available in large print and on cassette.

The Guild for the Blind

180 North Michigan Avenue #1700
Chicago, IL 60601-7463
Phone: 312-236-8569

Free monthly publication in large print and/or Braille that announces Guild programs and reprints information from local and national publications.

Jewish Braille Institute of America, Inc

110 East 30th Street
New York, NY 10016
Phone: 800-433-1531

www.jewishbraille.org

Circulating library of Judaica for the blind, visually impaired, and reading disabled, available in large print, Braille, and cassette. Publishes Jewish Braille Review and JBI Voice. Prayer books available in Hebrew and English; cassettes available in English, Hebrew, Yiddish, Russian, Hungarian, Romanian, French and German. Free of charge.

Library of Congress
National Library Service for the Blind
1291 Taylor St. NW
Washington, DC 20542
Phone: 800-424-8567

www.loc.gov.nls

Maintains a free talking book service that includes recorded books and magazines for all ages. Ask for your local area and how to apply.

Lutheran Braille Workers, Inc.
P. O. Box 5000
Yucaipa, CA 92399
Phone: 909-795-8977

www.lbwinc.org

Lutheran Braille Workers, Inc. is a non-profit ministry providing Braille and large print bibles and other Christian-related books free of charge to visually impaired adults and children all over the world in 40 different languages.

New York Times Large Type Weekly
229 West 43rd Street
New York, NY 10036
Phone: 800-631-2580

www.nytimes.com/nytstore/publications

Prepared by the editors of The Week in Review with many of the Times features including the NY Times crossword puzzle. Offers subscriptions to the weekly paper in large type ($35.10 for six months, $70.20 for twelve months).

Reader's Digest Large Type Edition
PO Box 262
Mt. Morris, IL 61054
Phone: 800-877-5293

www.rd.com

In addition to the regular monthly magazine, Reader's Digest Great Biographies, Condensed Books, and Bibles are also available in large type.

United States Blind Golfers Association
3094 Shamrock Street N.
Tallahassee, FL 32308-2735
Phone/FAX: 904-893-4511

www.blindgolf.com

Provides a quarterly newsletter, The Midnight Golfer Newsletter, containing information regarding golfing competitions for the blind or visually impaired.

Xavier Society for the Blind
154 East 23rd Street
New York, NY 10010-4595
Phone: 212 473-7800

Publishes the bi-monthly Catholic Review in Braille, large print, and cassette tape. Has religious material and textbooks available in all three formats and maintains a free lending library. Offers Bible reading program.

References – Chapter Six

Ball K, Owsley C, Sloane ME, Roenker DL, Bruni JR. Visual attention problems as a predictor of vehicle crashes in older drivers. Invest Ophthalmol Vis Sci 1993; 34: 3110-3123.

Berdeaux GH, Nordmann JP, Colin E, Arnould B. Vision-related quality of life in patients suffering from age-related macular degeneration. Am J Ophthalmol 2005; 139: 271-279.

Brown, GC, Brown, MM, Sharma S. The Burden of Macular Degeneration. Proceedings of The Macula Society 28th Annual Scientific Program. Key Biscayne, Florida, February 24, 2005, p. 52.

Brown GC, Murphy RP. Visual symptoms associated with choroidal neovascularization: Photopsias and the Charles Bonnet syndrome. Arch Ophthalmol 1992; 110: 1251-1256.

Holroyd S, Rabins PV, Finkelstein D, Nicholson MC, Chase GA, Wisniewski SC. Visual hallucinations in patients with macular degeneration. Am J Psychiatry 1992; 149: 1701-1706.

Hu PS, Young J. 1990 Nation Wide Personal Transportation Survey: Demographic special report: Oakridge National Laboratories; 1994.

Knudtson MD, Klein BEK, Klein R, Cruickshanks KJ, Lee KE. Age-related eye disease, quality of life, and functional activity. Arch Ophthalmol 2005; 123: 807-814.

Menon, GJ. Complex visual hallucinations in the visually impaired: A structured history-taking approach. Arch Ophthalmol 2005; 123: 349-355.

National Safety Council. Crash Facts; 1992. Chicago; 1992.

Owsley C, McGwin G Jr. Visual impairment and driving. Surv Ophthalmol 1999; 43: 535-550

Rosenbloom AA Jr. Care of the visually impaired elderly patient. In: Rosenbloom AA Jr,. Morgan MW, eds. Vision and Aging: General and Clinical Perspectives. New York: Professional Press Books; 1986: 343.

Rosenbloom S. The mobility needs of the elderly. In: Committee for the Study on Improving Mobility and Safety for Older Persons. Transportation in an aging society: Improving mobility and safety for older persons. Washington, DC: Transporation Research Board, National Research Council, 1988.

Rosenbloom S. Transportation needs of the elderly population. Clin Geriatr Med 1993; 9: 297-310.

Rovner BW, Casten RJ, Tasman WS. Effect of depression on vision function in age-related macular degeneration. Arch Opthalmol 2002; 120: 1041-1044.

Silver JH, Gould ES, Irvine D, Cullinan TR. Visual acuity at home and in eye clinics. Trans Ophthalmol Soc UK 1978; 98: 262-266.

Submacular Surgery Trials Research Group. Patients' perceptions of the value of current vision: Assessment of preference values among patients with subfoveal choroidal neovascularization – the Submacular Surgery Trials Vision Preference Value Scale: SST Report No. 6. Arch Ophthalmol 2004; 122: 1856-1867.

Chapter 8: Sustaining safe mobility in older drivers. In: Highway Safety Strategies for Iowa. Last modified 11/20/2002. Accessed at: http://www.iowasms.org/toolbox/chapter08.pdf on September 23, 2005.

Chapter Seven
The Future

Research into the cause and treatment for AMD is progressing rapidly. The field of molecular genetics has given us powerful tools to figure out why some people get a disease whereas others don't. Already a number of genes associated with AMD have been discovered, and we believe that most of the rest will be discovered in the next five years. The genes are like the blueprints use by the cells to make necessary proteins or other molecules in the body. Once we know which gene (blueprint) is abnormal, we can determine what protein is made by the cells using this blueprint. Presumably this protein will also be abnormal and not function like it should, thus causing macular degeneration. So we'll know where the weakness is, the crack in the concrete, so to speak, which leads to problems later in life. One way to prevent vision loss would be to try to strengthen the weak area.

This is already happening. For instance, the discovery of mutations in the H factor of the complement system (see Chapter 2) clearly showed that inflammation was involved in many cases of AMD. Now scientists are concentrating on inflammation and trying to figure out how to control the runaway inflammation involved in AMD.

Right now we lump all patients with AMD together when we do clinical trials. The results of any given trial are the average of all the patients in the trial. But what really happens is that some patients in the trial do spectacularly well whereas others don't. The reason for the difference is probably that AMD is not a single disease but is made up of many diseases that look similar. The patients who do well in a particular trial may have one type of AMD, and the patients who do poorly may have another type. Therefore, the conclusions drawn from the results of the trial may help one group of AMD sufferers a lot, but do nothing or even harm other groups. Once we have identified all the genes involved in AMD, we can test individual patients and know which type of AMD they have. We will then be able to figure out what treatment works best for them. We can also put an abnormal gene in mice and literally have thousands of "patients" with that type of AMD. We can then quickly test a new treatment to see if it works for that type of AMD at a fraction of the cost of clinical trials using human patients.

There have been great advances in the treatment of the wet form of the disease. For many years, pharmaceutical companies have been working on drugs which cause new blood vessels to regress. These drugs were originally developed to eradicate cancer by destroying the blood vessels that feed the tumor, but now we know that at least some of them also control the new blood vessels in the wet form of AMD. Visudyne®, Macugen®, and Retaane® have slowed the progression of the disease. Now drugs like Avastin® and Lucentis® actually improve the vision of many patients with the wet form of AMD. In a few years we have gone from the sad situation where most patients who have wet AMD lose a lot of vision to one where most patients remain stable or even get better vision with treatment.

In five years, you'll be able to get a blood test that evaluates your DNA and determines your risk of AMD, and of many other diseases, for that matter. You'll know whether you're at high risk of AMD and also know which type of the disease you're most likely to get. In five or maybe ten years, we will know which specific steps you should take to lower the risk of vision loss. For example, one type of AMD may respond particularly well to antioxidants and zinc supplements whereas another type may not. Another type may respond to anti-inflammatory agents or cholesterol-lowering agents. Once we know the gene we'll find the cause of the AMD. Once we know the cause, we can design a treatment to stop it or at least slow it down.

In five years, we'll probably have drugs that prevent or at least lower the risk of developing the wet form of AMD. It would be best to prevent the blood vessels from ever occurring, but the treatments for the abnormal blood vessels, if they sneak through our preventive treatment, will be better too. Most people who are at risk will be able to sharply lower this risk through lifestyle changes, diet and supplements, and medications. AMD doesn't usually cause vision loss until a patient is in their seventies. New treatments don't necessarily have to completely cure the disease, just postpone it for twenty years.

Some people, though, will have the type of AMD which causes loss of vision at a relatively early age (55 to 60 years old) for this disease. Often this "bad" form runs in families and is due to a severe genetic defect. Even if these patients do everything they can to reduce their risk, they may be able to postpone vision loss only for five or ten years. These patients may be candidates for gene transplantation. We are already transplanting genes into monkey retinas at The University of Iowa, and other research groups are working feverishly on similar projects. We are concentrating now on diseases, such as severe retinitis pigmentosa, which can cause total blindness at younger ages than when AMD occurs. But once the techniques are perfected, it should not be a big jump to transplanting normal genes in place of defective genes in patients who we know are going to get severe AMD.

You can do a lot to advance research in AMD. You can volunteer to participate in clinical trials. You can donate your eyes for research after you die. If you have a strong family history of the disease, you can round up family members to be examined and have their blood taken for genetic screening. And you can give money to research. There are many very bright scientists and doctors in the world working on this disease. There is no lack of brainpower or ideas. It's always a lack of money that slows research. More money means more research and new treatments. We will list agencies and institutions at the end of this book who are active in AMD research. In almost all of the cases, your donation is tax deductible. You can also write your representatives in Congress and urge them to increase funding for medical research and especially for research in AMD. Medical research pays for itself over and over again in the reducing cost of illness and improving quality of life. It is a terrific investment in the future.

Chapter Eight
What Should You Do Now?
How to Keep up on the Latest in AMD

The first thing we suggest you do is determine your risk. If you have a parent or sibling with AMD, then your risk is higher for the disease. But not having a relative with the disease doesn't mean that you will never get AMD. You should have your eyes examined by an eye doctor. I would tell the doctor that you wish to know if you have any signs of AMD. The doctor must dilate your pupils to get a good look at your retina. Many eye doctors will be willing to take a picture of your maculas if you wish. If the doctor sees any medium- or large-size drusen, then you're at risk of vision loss. We are not sure whether having a few tiny drusen means you have the disease or not.

The Age-related Eye Disease Study (AREDS) broke down the risk of vision loss in terms of whether or not there was the presence of one large druse and whether or not there was pigmentation. Experts examined all of the photographs in the study and developed a point system to estimate the risk of developing advanced AMD over 5 years. The presence of one large drusen in an eye was one point. If both eyes had large drusen, that was two points. The presence of pigmentation in the macula was also one point and if it was present in both eyes, again, it was two points. That means a patient could have up to a total of four points. Please go back to Chapter One to see photos of patients who have large drusen and pigmentation.

The risk of developing severe AMD over the next five years in at least one eye was 0.5 percent in patients who had neither large drusen nor pigmentation in either eye (zero points). The risk was 3 percent over five years for patients who had one point; 12 percent for patients who had two points; 25 percent for patients with three points; and 50 percent for patients who had four points. That is why we suggested in Chapter One that you ask your doctor whether you have any large drusen or pigmentation in either eye.

This simplified point system doesn't directly address those with medium-size drusen. Basically if a patient has a few medium-size drusen, the risk is low. If the patient has a lot of medium-size drusen, the risk becomes similar to a patient with a large druse.

Patients with only a few small drusen are at low risk for severe AMD at least for the next five years and probably for much longer. Many of these patients never develop AMD.

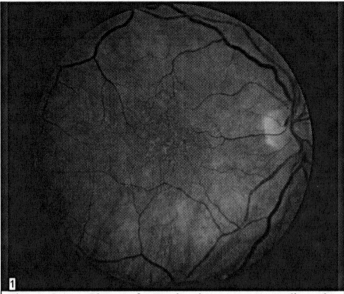

Figure 8-1A- Photo of macula shows many medium-size drusen. Patient is at risk for severe AMD.

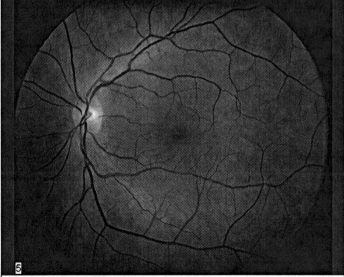

Figure 8-1B- Wide-field photo of a macula with only a few small drusen. Risk of severe AMD is very low.

If you have signs of early AMD, I suggest you do the following:

1. Stop smoking. There are new drugs that can help you quit. You should see your family doctor who will be delighted to help you.

2. Take supplements following the AREDS daily doses: vitamin C, 500 milligrams; beta-carotene, 15 milligrams or about 28,000 IU; vitamin E, 400 IU; zinc as zinc oxide, 80 milligrams; and copper, 2 milligrams.

3. Consider taking lutein, 10 milligrams; zeaxanthine, 2 milligrams; and omega-3 fish oil, 1.5 grams a day. Better yet, eat a diet rich in these nutrients, with colored fruits and vegetables every day and baked or broiled fish twice a week (see Chapter Four). The National Eye Institute is sponsoring a new study called AREDS II which will test whether these supplements are helpful. We recommend you join this study if possible because then you'll be kept up on the latest information.

4. There are a few small studies which showed that low selenium levels might be associated with AMD. Most Americans, however, get enough selenium in the diet so we don't recommend supplementation. Daily doses of over 400 micrograms of selenium can be toxic. Selenium is a heavy metal and should not be considered an herbal supplement.

Controlled studies have shown that bilberry doesn't improve night vision. There is no evidence or reason to believe that it would be helpful in people with AMD. One AMD supplement contains chromium but there is no evidence that supplementation with this metal is helpful in patients with AMD.

5. Lose weight until you're in the normal range of fat percentage for your gender and age. This is especially important if the fat is concentrated around your belly.

6. If your cholesterol is high, ask your doctor to prescribe you a drug from the "statin" group.

7. Obtain an Amsler grid from your eye doctor. Call promptly if you notice any blurred or distorted vision that lasts more than a few hours.

8. If you have suffered vision loss, go to a good low vision clinic. Be sure to tell your doctor if you have any signs of depression. Remain active and don't isolate yourself.

Special Concerns:

1. What kind of doctor should I see if I'm worried about age-related macular degeneration?

AMD is a common disease so the vast majority of optometrists (doctors of optometry who graduated from an optometry school) or comprehensive ophthalmologists (medical doctors who graduated from a medical school and then took an ophthalmology residency) should be able to diagnose the disease. Therefore, either of these doctors should be able to diagnose AMD.

If you need treatment, however, you probably should see a retinal specialist. A retinal specialist has had an additional one to two years of advanced training (called a fellowship) in the field of retina after he or she has completed a residency in ophthalmology.

2. How can I tell if my eye doctor knows what he or she is doing?

The knowledge you've gained in this book should help you be able to tell whether your eye doctor is competent. To summarize what was discussed in Chapter One: Your eye doctor should be able to tell you whether he sees drusen in your eyes; he should be able to tell you whether they're large drusen and whether you have any other signs of AMD, such as pigmentation, atrophy, or neovascularization. He should also know about the results of the AREDS trial.

3. When do I need a referral?

If your eye doctor fails the above tests; in other words, if he or she bumbles and stumbles around when you ask if he sees drusen and what size they are, you should see someone else. Most comprehensive ophthalmologists and many optometrists are competent at diagnosing dry AMD. Your doctor should be able to explain clearly why you're losing vision and show you a picture of your eye.

You need a referral to a retinal specialist any time you lose vision rapidly or have distorted vision. You also need a referral if you don't feel comfortable about what the doctor tells you. Some patients worry that they'll offend their doctors if they ask for a referral. However, doctors shouldn't feel offended and if they do, it's probably a sign that you need to get another doctor anyway because this one is too arrogant. You must be your own advocate.

4. How can you tell whether the retinal specialist knows what he or she is doing?

The answer to this is pretty much the same as for the optometrist or comprehensive ophthalmologist. The retinal specialist should clearly explain to you why you are losing vision. He should show you the pictures of your maculas. He should tell you whether you have the wet form of the disease. In general, if you have new blood vessels, he should offer you one of the treatments listed in Chapter Five. If he doesn't, he should explain why and recommend that he see you again in a month or two.

5. Are there super-specialists in the field of AMD?

There are experts in the field of AMD, but generally they will not offer you much more than your local retinal specialist. You can certainly travel to see an expert in AMD. These days, however, it might be easier to send him or her digital photographs of your eyes. Usually the specialist will be able to tell from your history and the pictures whether you are on the right track with your treatment.

Keeping Up on the Latest: The Internet

(by Patricia Duffel, R.Ph., M.A., Librarian, Department of Ophthalmology and Visual Sciences, The University of Iowa)

We believe that individuals with AMD should have ready access to the internet. The internet is a great tool for learning and is the best source for someone to find out the latest information about AMD. The internet is open to everyone and therein lies its strength and weakness. It's freely available for all of us, and at the same time anyone can write pretty much anything on it. Therefore, one needs to be a savvy user to separate the wheat from the chaff or from the utter nonsense. Here are some tips for using the internet as a reference tool:

Don't Believe Everything You Read

Keep in mind that not all information is written by a qualified expert. No one regulates information on the internet. There is no guarantee that the information you find is accurate or up-to-date. However, it is possible to find accurate information on the internet or in print. Below we give you tips on how to evaluate the credibility and accuracy of information found on the internet.

Use Information Wisely

It can be hard to judge the accuracy and credibility of medical information. Even people with medical backgrounds sometimes find this task daunting. Magazines, television news, radio talk shows, newspapers, websites, friends, relatives, and acquaintances may or may not give you accurate information. Here are some tips to help you decide what information to believe:

- Consider the source. Was the article published in a peer-reviewed journal, where articles are reviewed by other qualified members of the profession for accuracy and reliability? Do medical experts serve as editors and review articles? Does a website have medical editors or consultants?

- Google the authors. Check the author's credentials by looking up his or her affiliations, whether and where he or she attended college and medical school, and lists of his or her other publications.

- Who is responsible for the website? There should be accountability for the information displayed or printed. Credentials should be clearly displayed on the website. If the authors, organization, and credentials are missing, consider this a red flag. Anyone can set up a home page and claim anything.

- Government agencies, health foundations, and professional organizations are generally the best sources for unbiased material. The addresses of these websites usually end in .gov for government or .org for organization. Such groups would include the National Institutes of Health, the National Eye Institute, the National Advisory Eye Council, the American Academy of Ophthalmology, the American Academy of Optometry, and Research to Prevent Blindness, Inc. The American Heart Association and US Department of Agriculture have good information on nutrients in foods.

- Educational institutions (which have websites with addresses ending in .edu) usually provide reliable health-related information. However, you should be aware that these institutions are also competing for patients and research money so they may exaggerate the value of new treatments that are available at their institution.

- Websites with addresses ending in .com are commercial sites designed to sell you something. Their information is suspect. Some commercial sites get around this by calling themselves an organization. For instance, "The American Academy for the Treatment of Macular Degeneration.org" – it sounds good, doesn't it? I just made it up. Anyone else could do the same and use a credible-sounding name and a .org designation to sell you something unproven. So you have to dig a little beyond just the name of the website to check the credentials of whoever's responsible for it

- Check for references. Is the information given in the website just opinion or fact? Are the claims backed up by the research literature? Look for a list of references at the end of the source. Information that's backed up by other medical professionals and researchers is more likely to be accurate.
- Compare several different resources on the same topic. Check two or three independent sources to see whether the information or advice is similar.
- Ask yourself whether the information or advice seems to contradict what you've learned from your doctor or from reading. If so, talk to your doctor to clarify the differences in the information.
- Ask yourself if the information or advice "rings true." Does it make sense? Is the information plausible? Does it jive with your common sense, or does it sound too sensational?
- Be cautious about making decisions based on information printed in newspapers and magazines or broadcast on television, radio, or news websites. Most reporters are journalists, not medical experts. Reporters may exaggerate a bit to attract more readers or viewers. Medical facts and statistics can be misunderstood, misinterpreted, misrepresented, or incomplete.
- Check to see whether the reporter cites a source for his information and includes the credentials of the persons cited.
- Is it an advertisement? Don't trust medical product advertisements claiming miracle cures or spectacular results. Even if nothing is being sold on a website, ask yourself if the host of the site has an interest in promoting a particular product or service.
- Be cautious when using information heard at social gatherings, found on electronic bulletin boards, or during "chat" sessions with others. Testimonials and personal stories are based on one person's experience rather than on objective facts or proven

medical research. Commercial sites often use testimonials from grateful users of their product instead of solid scientific information. There's no way to judge whether their stories are true or whether other customers have had a similar or a very different outcome.

Helpful and Accurate Websites

MedlinePlus.gov will direct you to information that helps answer health questions. MedlinePlus brings together authoritative information from NLM, the National Institutes of Health (NIH), and other government agencies and health-related organizations. MedlinePlus also has extensive information about drugs, an illustrated medical encyclopedia, interactive patient tutorials, and latest health news. The MedlinePlus Encyclopedia entry for AMD is at http://www.nlm.nih.gov/medlineplus/ency/article/001000.htm.

The list of AMD sites is at
http://www.nlm.nih.gov/medlineplus/maculardegeneration.html

The National Institutes of Health, NIH Senior Health site has information on Macular Degeneration at
http://nihSeniorHealth.gov/AgeRelatedMacularDegeneration/toc.html

The National Eye Institute has "Age-Related Macular Degeneration: What you should know." at
http://www.nei.nih.gov/health/maculardegen/armd_facts.asp as well as "Don't Lose Sight of Age-Related Macular Degeneration" at
http://www.nei.nih.gov/health/maculardegen/armd_risk.asp

You can browse a list of Macular Degeneration Trials at Clinical Trials.gov http://tinyurl.com/7784x

The Department of Transportation has information about driving with macular degeneration at
http://www.nhtsa.dot.gov/people/injury/olddrive/Driving_macular/

The Healthfinder database also has a list of government Macular Degeneration sites at http://www.healthfinder.gov/Scripts/SearchContext.asp?topic=513.

Other good websites:

The American Academy of Ophthalmology, http://www.aao.org/

The American Academy of Optometry, http://www.aaopt.org/

The American Macular Degeneration Foundation, http://www.macular.org/

The American Optometric Association, http://www.aoanet.org/

The Association for Macular Diseases, http://www.macula.org/

Foundation Fighting Blindness, http://www.blindness.org/

Lighthouse International, http://www.lighthouse.org/

The Macular Degeneration Foundation, http://www.eyesight.org/

The Macular Degeneration Partnership, http://www.amd.org/site/PageServer

The National Eye Institute, http://www.nei.nih.gov/

Prevent Blindness American, http://www.preventblindness.org/

Research to Prevent Blindness, http://www.rpbusa.org/

United States Department of Agriculture, http://www.usda.gov, particularly "What's in food?" http://tinyurl.com/aucg7

American Dietetic Association, http://www.eatright.org/

References – Chapter Eight

Age-Related Eye Disease Study Research Group. The Age-Related Eye Disease Study Severity Scale for age-related macular degeneration: AREDS Report No. 17. Arch Ophthalmol 2005; 123: 1484-1498.

Federal Citizen Information Center. "How to Find Medical Information." 2005; Cited Nov 11, 2005. Available from http://www.pueblo.gsa.gov/cic_text/health/med-info/med-info.htm#how8.

Mitchell P, Foran S. Age-Related Eye Disease Study Severity Scale and Simplified Severity Scale for age-related macular degeneration. Arch Ophthalmol 2005; 123: 1598-1599.

Pirbhai A, Sheidow T, Hooper P. Prospective evaluation of digital non-stereo color fundus photography as a screening tool in age-related macular degeneration. Am J Ophthalmol 2005; 139: 455-461.

A Final Word

We hope that you have found this book useful. Age-related macular degeneration is a serious disease but there are many things you can do right now to save your sight. And the future is looking very clear and bright. If you have any questions, you can contact us at:

MedRounds Publications Inc. http://www.medrounds.org/amd/

University of Iowa Center for Macular Degeneration
http://www.c4md.org/

Glossary and Index

Absorptive lenses: Glasses with tinted lenses used to absorb sunlight and prevent it from entering the eye. They are used to treat photophobia and to increase contrast; 101.

Age-Related Eye-Disease Study (AREDS): A large randomized study sponsored by the National Eye Institute which proved that supplementation with vitamins C, E, beta-carotene, zinc, and copper reduce the progression of AMD; 39.

Age-Related Eye Disease Study II (AREDS II): A study just started that will test whether supplementation with lutein and zeaxanthin as well as omega-3 polyunsaturated fatty acids will reduce the progression of AMD. AREDS II will also test if lower doses of beta-carotene and zinc are as effective as higher doses in reducing the risk of progression to severe AMD; 44.

Age-Related Macular Degeneration (AMD): A disease of the central retina first manifested by drusen in the macula. The disease can progress to atrophy of the outer retina or choroidal neovascularization.

   a. Dry AMD: includes drusen and atrophy; 8.

   b. Neovascular or wet AMD: blood vessels have grown from the choroid under the RPE and retina. These blood vessels leak fluid and blood and cause scarring; 10.

Alcon: The pharmaceutical and instrument company that makes anecortave acetate, or Retaane®.

Amsler grid: A checkerboard pattern of vertical and horizontal lines with a fixation dot in the middle. Used by patients to check for distortion or blank spots in their central vision; 10, 12.

ANCHOR: The acronym for the Anti-VEGF Antibody for the Treatment of Predominantly Classic Choroidal Neovascularization in AMD trial. This is an ongoing trial testing whether Lucentis® prevents vision loss in patients with AMD who have the classic type of choroidal neovascularization; 72.

Anecortave acetate: The generic name for Retaane®; 73.

Anecortave Acetate Risk Reduction Trial (AART): A trial underway in which patients who have AMD and neovascularization in one eye only are randomized to receive either 15 mg of anecortave acetate, 30 mg of anecortave acetate, or a placebo. The injections are given under the outside tissue on top of the eye every six months. The study is designed to determine if anecortave acetate reduces the risk of neovascularization in the second eye; 75.

Angular magnification: Increasing the apparent size of an object through the use of single or multiple lens systems, such as hand magnifiers or binoculars; 95.

Antioxidants: Vitamins and other molecules that eliminate reactive oxygen species and protect cells from damage; 37, 38, 40, 41, 48.

Atrophy: The most common cause of vision loss in AMD, Sometimes also called retinal pigment epithelial or geographic atrophy. Atrophy is a thinning and loss of tissue in the outer retina and retinal pigment epithelium which allows the underlying choroidal vessels to become visible; 8.

Avastin®: An antibody against vascular endothelial growth factor whose generic name is bevacizumab. Avastin is used to treat metastatic colon cancer and is the parent molecule of Lucentis®; 72.

Beta-carotene: A pigment found in fruits and vegetables which is converted to vitamin A in the body; 38, 40, 42, 43, 45, 46, 48, 51.

Bevacizumab: The generic name for Avastin®.

Bilberry: A perennial, ornamental shrub with berries (also called huckleberries in the United States). French researchers found that the jam from bilberries increased night vision of pilots in the Royal Air Force. Subsequent studies didn't confirm these findings. There is no evidence that bilberry helps AMD; 53, 55.

Binocular vision: Vision that uses both eyes to form a combined image in the brain which results in three-dimensional vision.

Bruch's membrane: A layered membrane that lies between the choriocapillaris and retinal pigment epithelium; 3-4.

Carotenoids: A large family of pigments synthesized by plants and play an important role in maintaining health. Beta-carotene is one carotenoid that is metabolized to vitamin A. Lutein and zeaxanthin are other carotenoids that are found in the macula; 39, 49.

Cataract surgery: Its effect on AMD; 21, 32-33.

Charles Bonnet Syndrome: Formed hallucinations caused by the brain in someone who has lost vision in both eyes; 108.

Choriocapillaris: Fine blood vessels in the inner choroid that lie next to Bruch's membrane and are responsible for bringing nutrients to the RPE and outer retina; 84.

Choroid: The vascular, very middle layer of the eye. The choroid lies between the inner retina and the outer sclera of the eye; 3, 7, 8, 10, 16, 21.

Choroidal neovascularization: The ingrowth of abnormal blood vessels from the choroid beneath the retinal pigment epithelium and retina in AMD and other diseases; 40, 61, 65, 70, 72, 73, 74

Chromium: A trace mineral in the diet. Chromium insufficiency may cause problems with glucose metabolism. There is no evidence that supplementation with chromium is helpful in AMD; 54, 56.

Classic choroidal neovascularization: New blood vessels that fill early with fluorescein dye and then leak profusely. Classic neovascularization typically progresses more rapidly than occult neovascularization; 65, 72.

Complications of AMD Prevention Trial (CAPT): A trial nearing completion. Patients who had drusen in both eyes were randomized to receive light laser treatment in one eye. This was done to stimulate the resorption of the drusen and preserve vision, but results are not yet known; 74, 75.

Cone cells: Specialized receptors in the outer retina that absorb light and convert it into a chemical signal; 3, 6-8.

Contrast sensitivity testing: A test that measures the ability to detect subtle differences in grayness. It is used to assess quality of vision as opposed to standard acuity charts which look at quantity of vision. Contrast sensitivity may be a better test of visual functioning in real-world situations than standard visual acuity charts which are high-contrast black on white; 92, 103.

Control group: A group of patients who are not receiving the treatment being tested in a clinical trial. This group is compared to the treatment group to see if there is a difference in the outcomes.

Corticosteroids: Drugs analogous to cortisol which decrease inflammation; 67-68.

C-Reactive Protein: A protein produced by the liver that can be measured in the blood. Elevated levels indicate inflammation in the body; 20, 50.

Docosahexaenoic acid (DHA): One of the omega-3 fatty acids found in fish and thought to reduce inflammation and the risk of heart disease and AMD; 47, 49.

Drusen (plural), Druse (singular): Collections of abnormal material beneath the retinal pigment epithelium that are the first clinical signs of AMD. Drusen are round and appear yellow on clinical examination; 6-8.

Drusen have been divided into the following sizes for research purposes:.

a. Small drusen – smaller than 63 microns in size; 5.

b. Medium drusen – 63-125 microns in size; 8.

c. Large drusen – larger than 125 microns in size; 5.

Dry AMD: The macula has drusen and atrophy of photoreceptors and RPE but no new blood vessels in distinction to wet or neovascular AMD; 8.

Eicosapentaenoic acid (EPA): One of the omega-3 fatty acids found in fish and thought to reduce inflammation and the risk of heart disease and AMD; 47, 49.

Electric stimulation: A treatment that has been touted for the treatment of AMD but probably has no benefit; 83.

Endophthalmitis: An infection inside the eye that is usually bacterial and very serious; 70.

Epidemiology: The study of which factors affect the presence or absence of a disease; 28.

Eyetech: The company that makes and sells Macugen®.

Factor H; see H Factor.

Fibulin: A family of genes that code for structural proteins found in the eye and elsewhere in the body. A small percentage of patients with AMD have defects in the fibulin genes; 19.

FOCUS: The acronym for RhuFab V2 Ocular Treatment Combining the Use of Visudyne™ to Evaluate Safety. This study showed that Lucentis combined with Visudyne was more effective for the treatment of the wet form of AMD than Visudyne alone; 71.

Fluorescein angiography (FFA): A photographic test commonly used to image the retinal and choroidal blood vessels. A small amount of fluorescein dye is injected into an arm vein. The dye circulates through the bloodstream and flows into the blood vessels of the eye. Special filters are used to stimulate the dye and the images are captured on film or digitally; 14.

Genentech: The biotech company that manufactures Avastin® and Lucentis®.

Glaucoma: An eye disease that causes progressive damage to the optic nerve, usually from elevated intraocular pressure. Corticosteroids used as an adjunct treatment in AMD can cause elevations of the intraocular pressure and glaucoma; 68.

H-factor, Factor H: A protein involved in the regulation of inflammation in the body. Abnormalities in this protein have been associated with AMD implying that inflammation is associated with the disease; 20.

Hypertension: High blood pressure; 29, 32.

Internet: How to use wisely; 134.

Kenalog®: The brand name for the corticosteroid, triamcinolone acetonide. The drug can be injected around or into the eye and has been used along with Visudyne® for the treatment of wet AMD; 67.

Laser: An acronym that stands for Light Amplification through Stimulated Emitted Radiation or, in practical terms, a strong beam of light of the same color. The light does not diverge (spread apart) so it can be used for aiming devices or burning tissue; 63, 74, 79, 82.

Legal blindness: A definition developed by the Social Security Administration to determine eligibility for benefits or services in the United States. It is defined as best corrected visual acuity, with contact lenses or spectacles, in the better seeing eye, of 20/200 or less or a visual field restriction of 20 degrees or less, at its widest extent, in the better eye; 118.

Linolenic acid: Actually alpha-linolenic acid (ALA). ALA is found in nuts and some oils and converted to eicosapentaenoic acid (EPA) and docosahexaenoic acid (DHA) which are essential fatty acids that reduce inflammation and the risk of heart disease and AMD; 47.

Linoleic acid: One of the essential omega-6 fatty acids. Found in vegetable oils and animal fat. The western diet is thought to contain too much linoleic acid and too high a ratio of linoleic (omega-6) to linoleic (omega-3) fatty acids. AMD patients should reduce consumption of linoleic acid; 46.

Lucentis®: Generic name is ranibizumab. An antibody to vascular endothelial growth factor that has been proven to reduce vision loss and even to increase vision in patients with neovascular AMD; 70.

Lutein: A carotenoid found in high quantities in the macula; 43.

Macugen®: Generic name is pegaptanib. A molecule that inhibits one form of vascular endothelial growth factor. Has been found to reduce vision loss, when compared to no treatment, in patients with the neovascular form of AMD; 69.

Macula: The central part of the retina that allows for detailed vision; 3.

Macular Photocoagulation Study (MPS): A series of randomized controlled trials that proved thermal laser preserved vision in patients with the wet form of AMD; 17.

Macular translocation: A surgery during which the retina is detached and moved to an area of RPE not involved with new blood vessels as a treatment for neovascular AMD. There are two types:

a. Limited macular translocation – the retina is not cut but detached and pushed inferiorly with a gas bubble; 80.

b. Three hundred and sixty degree translocation – the retina is cut at the periphery and the retina is rotated to a new position; 81.

MARINA: The acronym for the Minimally classic/occult trial of the Anti-VEGF antibody Ranibizumab In the treatment of Neovascular AMD. This was the trial in which ranibizumab (Lucentis®) improved the vision at one-year in patients with the wet form of AMD compared to patients who had received sham injections; 71.

Metamorphopsia: Distortion in vision caused by fluid beneath or in the retina typically seen as a straight line looking bent. It is a common first symptom of neovascular AMD; 61.

Microscopic spectacles: High-powered convex lenses that magnify objects that are held close to the eye. The lenses are usually mounted into eyeglasses and prescribed for one eye only.

MIRA-1: The acronym for the Multicenter Investigation of Rheophoresis for AMD. Patients with AMD are randomized so that two-thirds of them receive rheophoresis and one-third receive a sham treatment. Results are expected in early 2006; 84.

Neovacular AMD: See wet AMD.

Novartis: The drug company that makes and sells verteporfin for Visudyne® treatment.

Occult choroidal neovascularization: This type of abnormal blood vessels fills more slowly with fluorescein than classic neovascularization and leaks less. Occult neovascularization often doesn't have a sharp boundary like classic neovascularization and tends to progress slower.

Obesity: Twenty to thirty percent above ideal body weight; 30, 37.

Omega-3 poly-unsaturated fatty acids: A group of fatty acids that include linolenic acid, DHA, and EPA which are helpful to reduce the risk of heart disease and AMD; 45, 49.

Omega-6 fatty acids: A group of fatty acids including linoleic acid. Although essential for body functions, they promote inflammation, heart disease, and AMD if taken in too high quantities compared to omega-3 fatty acids; 46, 47, 48

Optic Coherence Tomography (OCT): An imaging test using low-intensity laser to create a cross-section view of the retina. The test helps the eye doctor determine whether there is fluid beneath or within the retina; 77.

Optical device: Any system of lenses that enhances vision function.

Ophthalmologist: A medical doctor (MD or DO) who has graduated from a four-year medical school, then has completed a one-year internship and a three-year ophthalmology residency.

Optometrist: A doctor of optometry (OD) who has attended undergraduate school and then graduated from a four-year optometry school.

Pegaptanib: The generic name for Macugen®.

Photodynamic therapy (PDT): A treatment for wet AMD in which a light laser treatment is used to activate a dye and destroy the abnormal blood vessels. See Visudyne®; 64.

Photophobia: Light sensitivity to an uncomfortable degree; it usually indicates the presence of an ocular disorder or disease.

PIER: An acronym for A Phase IIIb, Multicenter, Randomized, Double-Masked, Sham Injection-Controlled Study of the Efficacy and Safety of Ranibizumab. It compares subjects with wet AMD who receive one of two doses of Lucentis® against those who receive sham injections. The Lucentis® is given once a month for three months and then only once every three months.

Pigment changes: Lines or dots of brown or black pigment in the macula which lie on the top of drusen. Pigment changes have been shown to be a risk factor for the progression to severe AMD; 4, 8, 9.

Placebo or placebo effect: The phenomenon that occurs because patients wish to get better. Many patients will perceive that they are improving even when given a treatment that has no effect. That is why a control group is necessary in clinical trials to compare to the group taking the new treatment; 54.

Radiation: A treatment that can use a variety of high energy particles that is usually used for the treatment of cancer. It has no benefit for the treatment of AMD; 82.

Randomized Controlled Trial: A study which tests a new treatment. Patients with a disease first enter they study and then are randomized (like flipping a coin) to receive the new treatment or a placebo treatment. The outcomes of the patients who receive the new treatment are then compared to the outcomes of the control patients who are receiving the placebo treatment; 62.

Ranibizumab: The generic name for Lucentis® which is an antibody that inhibits vascular endothelial growth factor and has been shown to be effective for treating the wet form of AMD; 70.

Reactive oxygen species: Molecules that form when oxygen reacts with light energy and which are destructive to cell membranes; 21, 38.

Relative distance magnification: Increasing the size of the image on the retina by bringing the object to be viewed closer to the eyes; 94.

Relative size magnification: Increasing the size of the image on the retina by increasing the size of the object to be viewed. Large print is an example of this; 94.

Retaane®: Brand name of anecortave acetate, a modified steroid that acts to prevent the growth of new blood vessels. It has been shown to reduce vision loss in the neovascular form of AMD; 73.

Retinal Pigment Epithelium (RPE): A layer of cells that lies between the photoreceptors and Bruch's membrane; 5.

Retinal Pigment Epithelial Detachment (RPED): An elevation of the RPE from Bruch's membrane seen mainly in AMD; 9.

Retinal specialist: An ophthalmologist who has completed one or two years of a retinal fellowship after an ophthalmology residency.

Rheophoresis: A technique analogous to renal dialysis in which the large proteins and lipids are removed from the serum. Rheophoresis has been touted as a treatment for AMD but there is little evidence that it's of any benefit; 84.

Scotoma: A blind spot in the vision. In AMD this can be due to atrophy, blood, or damage from neovascularization; 62.

Selenium: A trace mineral that is important in the function of the anti-oxidant enzyme, glutathione-peroxidase. Selenium is often included in vitamins for the eye but its value is unknown and there is a risk of toxicity if too much is taken; 39, 53, 55.

Smoking; 20, 21, 28, 29, 32, 36, 42, 44, 56.

Statin drugs: A large family of cholesterol-lowering drugs that may reduce the risk of AMD; 50, 57

Sunlight: And its affect on AMD; 30.

Subretinal Surgery Study (SST): A randomized controlled trial which showed no visual benefit of surgery in the wet form of AMD; 88.

Toll-like receptor: Defects in genes that code for this receptor have been found to be associated with AMD. The receptor is important for the functioning of macrophages which are involved in the removal of foreign matter from the body. The receptor also helps to remove the spent outer segments of cone cells so that they can be renewed; 20.

Thermal laser: A procedure wherein a strong laser beam is absorbed by pigment mainly in the RPE and converted to heat causing a destructive burn; 63.

Trans fats: Artificially hydrogenated vegetable oils that are bad for your eyes and heart. They are often found in margarine and other processed foods; 46.

Transpupillary thermal therapy (TTT): A treatment for neovascular AMD that involves slowly heating the abnormal vessels with an infrared laser. TTT has been replaced by more effective treatments; 81.

Triamcinolone acetonide: The generic name for Kenalog®.

Vascular endothelial growth factor (VEGF): A polypeptide that stimulates the growth of choroidal neovascularization in AMD; 69.

VERITAS: A study just underway. The acronym stands for VERteporfin (Visudyne®) plus two different dose regimens of Intravitreal Triamcinolone Acetonide versus Visudyne® plus intravitreal pegaptanib (Macugen®) in patients with Subfoveal choroidal neovascularization secondary to age-related macular degeneration.

Verteporfin: The dye used in Visudyne® treatment. It absorbs light and gives off free radicals which damage new blood vessels in AMD; 65, 79.

Visual acuity: A measure of sharpness of vision as related to the ability to distinguish the details and shapes of objects at a designated distance. Normally used as a measurement of central (macular) vision; 84, 92, 102, 103, 106.

Vision impairment: Any amount of vision loss that affects an individual's ability to perform the task of daily life resulting from damage or disease to the visual system or the result of the visual system not being formed correctly; 102, 105, 113.

Visudyne®: A type of photodynamic treatment that uses verteporfin as the excitable dye and has been proven to reduce vision loss in neovascular AMD compared to no treatment; 64.

Vitamins for AMD; 39, 41, 48, 49, 50.

Weight Loss: And its effect on AMD; 37.

Wet AMD: New blood vessels have grown and are leaking fluid or blood beneath and within the macula; also called neovascular AMD; in distinction to dry AMD; 10.

Zeaxanthin: A carotenoid pigment found in the macula; 43.